Rings of the Mind

eduardo padilla-diaz

The Rings of the Mind

Book 1 from the series: Modeling the Body-Mind

Eduardo Padilla-Diaz

Table of Contents

0. [Cover-1] *Rings of the Mind - Book 1 of the series: Modeling the Body-Mind.*
1. [TOC] *Thematics and Exploration Plan.*
2. [Conventions] *Considerations about revisions, references, TOCs, and Epilogs.*
3. [Abstract] *Brief about the incursions into the interior of the body, time, and mind.*
4. [Rings-1] *Explores from the origins of the universe to the atoms of all elements.*
5. [Rings-2] *Explores the molecular mind in the creation of all types of matter.*
6. [Rings-3] *Explores from the minds of molecular robots to the origins of life.*
7. [Rings-4] *Explores from the virtual mind to the human and external minds.*
8. [Vital Code] *Vital software is written with this code.*
9. [Memories-1] *Their physiology and where they are.*
10. [ATP Batteries] *Rechargeable molecular batteries that energize all cells.*
11. [ZPUs] *Molecular processors that execute bio-software resulting in chemical transformations.*
12. [Clocks] *All cells have a clock synchronized by a central clock in the brain.*
13. [Life] *Intelligent energy is transferred at the cellular level to create life at the human level.*
14. [Inconscience] *Aggregate functionality of all the minds below the virtual mind.*
15. [Objects of Interest] *The most transcendental concept in capturing useful sensory information.*
16. [Lingua Mentis] *An innate mechanism of a language is embedded in our brain.*

17. [Vocabularies] *Learning machines that transform sensations into cognitive particles.*
18. [Fields] *Sensory fields (visual, acoustic, etc.) that excite the sensors of our sensory centers.*
19. [MC-1] *The Motor Center 1 controls all our movements, from molecules to muscles.*
20. [VC-1] *The Visual Center 1 allows photons to show us visual reality.*
21. [Thinking-1] *Initiation to its models. Interfacing the Visual and Motor Centers to a Thinker.*
22. [Epilog-1] *Thematics of the next book in the series: The Width of the Present.*
23. [Copyrights] *List of copyright certificates that protect these works.*
24. [Dedication] *To my children: Mariana, Andres, and Camilo.*
25. [Back-cover-1] *Brief about the author Eduardo Padilla-Diaz and his works.*

Conventions

"Considerations about revisions, references, TOCs, and Epilogs."

2.1 Introduction

- In this work, the following conventions are followed:
1. Most of the paragraphs in the book are marked with icons that contain metadata (such as edition dates); at the reader level, they have the following meaning:
    - Final edition paragraph.
    - The paragraph contains a concept, proposal, or idea originated by the author Eduardo Padilla or a statement of something already existing but explained by the author in his own words.
2. Wikipedia is the preferred reference source throughout this book since it provides access to all references at no cost or membership ties. Furthermore, Wikipedia almost always extends to more authoritative reference sources. Since its creation in January 2001, Wikipedia has become the world's largest reference website, attracting more than one billion visitors monthly. It currently has more than fifty-nine million articles in more than 300 languages.
    - [wikipedia] wikipedia
3. The Tables of Contents and the Epilogs of every book of the series form a summary of the explorations.

Abstract

"Brief about the incursions into the interior of the body, time, and mind."

3.1 Introduction

- ◆ Reflections on this work:

- ◆ To understand the mind, we must first understand the body that hosts it. We need to know how the body is built, its parts, how they are created, and how they work. As we explore the gradual process of its construction, we will notice how the components of the mind emerge, and it will be easy for us to begin considering them. We will get to know why they are needed and how they are used, and when we finish building the body, we will start to understand what our mind is made of and, in part, how that wonder works.

- ◆ This work is a story of a daring adventure of exploration, which will take us through the confines of the human body. We'll explore everything from the universe's origins to the creation of all atoms, from the creation of molecules to the creation of all types of matter and structures, from the creation of molecular robots to the origins of human life. We'll explore: How rechargeable molecular batteries energize all cells. How molecular processors (ZPUs) execute bio-software, resulting in ultra-fast biochemical transformations that sustain an organism's metabolism. How all cells are synchronized. How intelligent energy is transferred at the cellular level to create life at the human level. How the objects of interest capture useful sensory information.

How the Lingua Mentis, an innate linguistic mechanism, is embedded in our brain. How learning machines transform sensations into cognitive particles. How Sensory fields (visual, acoustic, etc.) excite the sensors of our sensory centers. How the motor centers orchestrate all our movements. How the visual center allows photons to show us visual reality.

- This work includes a series of proposals for a thinking system. These proposals are presented progressively in several steps, assisted by models that make it easier to visualize how thinking works and its relationship with time, space, sensory centers, attention, motor centers, knowledge, imagination, intelligence, awareness, conscience, and reasoning.

- From the beginning of this work, I noticed the importance of considering the Nobel Prizes, awarded in appreciation to the discoveries that have helped elucidate the different forms of expression of matter and energy. That is why I redirected my effort and focused it on the areas where such awards were achieved, and that facilitated my research and gave me the confidence that I was on the right track in explaining how our body and mind work together. This work explicitly relates a significant part of its reflections with the discoveries of more than 80 Nobel Prize winners in physics, chemistry, physiology, and medicine.

- This work is the first of four books: The Rings of the Mind, The Width of the Present, Tokens and Words, and The Domains of the Conscience. It progressively presents the fundamental knowledge needed to understand and comprehend the models of thinking.

Rings-1

"Explores from the origins of the universe to the atoms of all elements."

4.1 Introduction

- Reflections on the mind part 1:
- Yes! The mind! that magical world in which we operate, where reality, time, and space can exist in all combinations of the real, virtual, emotional, and spiritual, where the conscience, subconscience, and inconscience operate concurrently to protect us from risk and the unexpected; where our 'Self' emerges, and makes us feel that we exist, lets us understand reality, allows us feel that others exist, lets us feel fantasies that fill us with hope and plenitude; where the laws that govern and describe it go beyond our understanding, and that is why until now we have not been able to understand it fully.
- We are going to propose a model of the mind based on a set of concentric mental rings, which form an ascending hierarchy, where the mental capacity of each ring is specific to its hierarchical level but which is formed based on the capabilities of the minds of all its inner rings.
  - That things build themselves is something we have to get used to. Yes! It does not fit into our reasoning that things self-multiply and self-modify to become what they should be, with precise and unimaginable functionality. The creation of all its parts occurs

harmoniously in parallel; minds creating minds, which are responsible for creating the human body, that incredible super robot - made by trillions of tiny robots - that carries us through our existence, where our minds, our self, and our conscience reside; with a capacity for knowledge, intelligence, imagination, and reasoning, that indicates that only the hand of God had to be behind that wonderful process.

- 🕐 Information structuring has allowed us to see the mind as a set of concentric rings, which encapsulate with great definition the functionality of the different types of minds and the types of matter that underlie them.

- 🕐 That is how we can begin to describe the mind as an aggregate operational state, which results from the contribution of several types of concentric minds, as indicated in the following model of the rings of the mind:

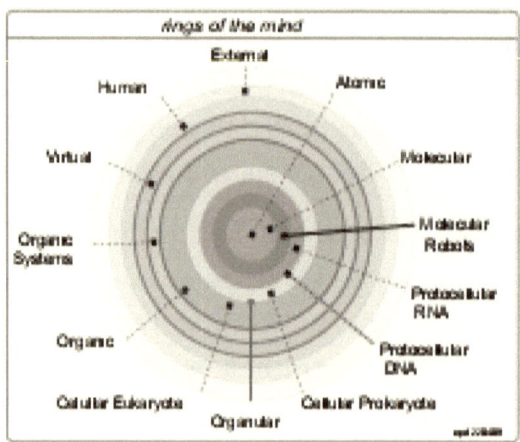

- 🕐 The incursion into minds lower than the atomic mind is excluded from this exploration; there is no doubt of their existence. I am still trying to find out how they would help me explain some of the enigmas still present in the minds of the upper rings.

4.2 Atomic Mind

- 🔹 The atomic mind exists in atoms to establish the laws governing all its particles' behavior. The main purpose of this mind is to guarantee that lasting and almost indestructible elements are created since they will be the foundation of everything that will be created in all the other rings of the mind. The hydrogen atom was formed first (H). It is the simplest and most abundant element since it constitutes 75% of the visible matter in the universe.
  - [atom] wikipedia

  - 🔹 Extrapolating the universe's expansion back several billion years, we reach a singular point where space and time lose meaning and is known as "the big bang singularity", which determines the universe's age.
    - [big bang] wikipedia [universe age adjusted to 26.7 billion years] openaccessgovernment.org

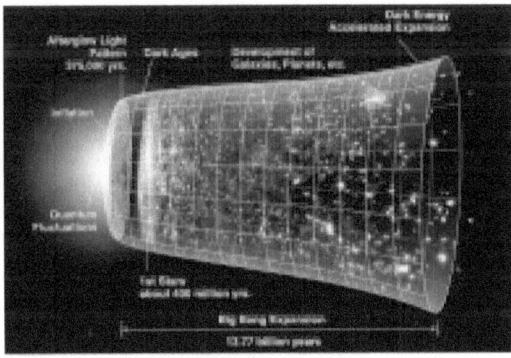

Fig. 4.1

- 🔹 The figure shows the cosmological epochs from the Big Bang to the present.
  - [cosmological epochs since the big bang] wikipedia [CMB Timeline 300 no WMAP] wikimedia

- ◉ In the first moments after the Big Bang, electrons were formed; then the protons and neutrons; then hydrogen nuclei were formed. Some of these nuclei combined to form helium and lithium, although in much smaller quantities.
  - [hydrogen]] [helium] wikipedia [how the first element was formed after the big bang]] astronomy.com

  - ◉ *The 1983 Nobel Prize in Physics was divided equally between Subramanyan Chandrasekhar "for his theoretical studies of the physical processes of importance for the structure and evolution of stars" and William Alfred Fowler "for his theoretical and experimental studies of the nuclear reactions of importance in the formation of chemical elements in the universe".*
    - [1983 Nobel Prize in Physics] nobelprize.org

- ◉ Stars are then formed, made primarily of hydrogen and helium, and they spend their lives generating their energy through the fusion of hydrogen; in which, for every 4 hydrogen atoms, one helium atom is formed, which has .7% less mass that is converted into energy, and that is what gives life and energy to the star.
  - [formation of stars] [fusion] wikipedia [the origin of the elements] youtube

- ◉ The following video, 'Origin of the Elements', by Edward Murphy, is an excellent presentation of how the elements that constitute all the matter in the universe are formed.
  - [origin of elements] youtube

- ◉ Through nuclear fusion, medium-sized stars like the sun produce certain elements, such as carbon, nitrogen, and oxygen. But when these stars

die, they become white dwarfs, and these elements are trapped in them.
    - [white dwarfs] wikipedia [origin of elements] youtube
- ⊙ ◈ The great stars, with masses 25 times greater than our sun, spend their lives fusing hydrogen into helium, helium into carbon, carbon into oxygen, and so on until they reach iron. Eventually, they become so massive, and their gravity is so strong that their core collapses; in the last two seconds of their life, they release so much energy, and all the other elements are made. The star explodes in a titanic explosion called a supernova, and most of its mass is launched into space to be used by future generations of stars.
    - [supernova] wikipedia [origin of elements] youtube

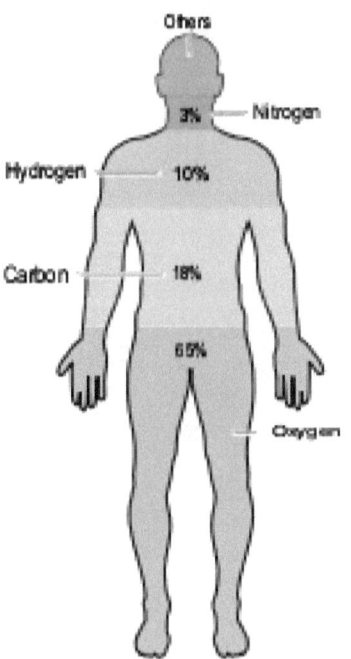

- ⊙ ◈ In our body, all the elements, be it carbon, nitrogen, and oxygen, did not come from a star like our sun but from a much larger star.
- ⊙ ◈ Note: 96% of our body mass is made up of just 4 elements: Oxygen 65%, Carbon 18%, Hydrogen 10%, and Nitrogen 3%.
    - [composition of the human body] wikipedia
- ⬤ ⇡◈ The atomic mind gives rise to the existence of the molecular mind.

eduardo padilla-diaz

Rings-2

"Explores the molecular mind in the creation of all types of matter."

5.1 Introduction

- Reflections on the rings of the mind (part 2):
- As we saw in the previous chapter, the atomic mind gave rise to the existence of the molecular mind, which is described below:

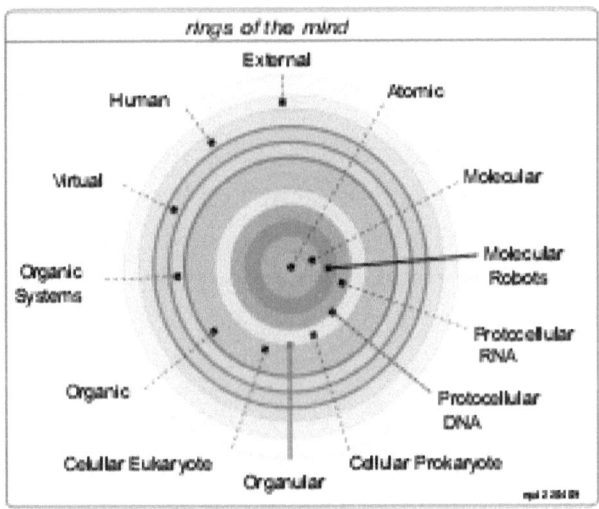

Fig. 5.1

5.2 Molecular Mind

- The molecular mind governs the behavior of atoms when they interact and form bonds between them. The purpose of this mind is to guarantee that stable and lasting bonds are created, allowing the creation of all types of

materials and structures that facilitate the storage and transfer of different types of energy and matter.
- [molecule] [bond] wikipedia

  - Molecules made from two atoms of the same element emerge, such as molecular hydrogen (H2) and molecular oxygen (O2):
    - Molecular hydrogen (H2) is the most common form of hydrogen and is very important in energy generation. It is the smallest molecule in the universe. Because it passes through plastic, it cannot remain in it.
      - [molecular hydrogen] yourwatermatters.com
    - The molecular oxygen (O2) is the one we breathe in the air.
      - [molecular oxygen] energyeducation.ca/encyclopedia
  - Then, molecules made of two elements emerge, also very useful, like water (H2O), methane (CH4), and ammonium (NH3); these, along with molecular hydrogen (H2), constitute in large part what could have been the atmosphere of the Earth in its origins.
    - [methane] [ammonium] wikipedia
  - Natural events that occurred more than ~3.5 billion years ago, similar to the one described below, would mark the genesis of macromolecules.
    - In 1953, the famous Miller-Urey experiment demonstrated that organic molecules could form spontaneously in the laboratory when a spark equivalent to lightning was applied to a group of gases, which simulated what the Earth's atmosphere could be like in its origins. The gases used were water (H2O) in gaseous state, methane (CH4), ammonium (NH3), and molecular hydrogen (H2). The figure shows a diagram of the Miller-Urey's experiment:

- [miller-urey experiment] wikipedia

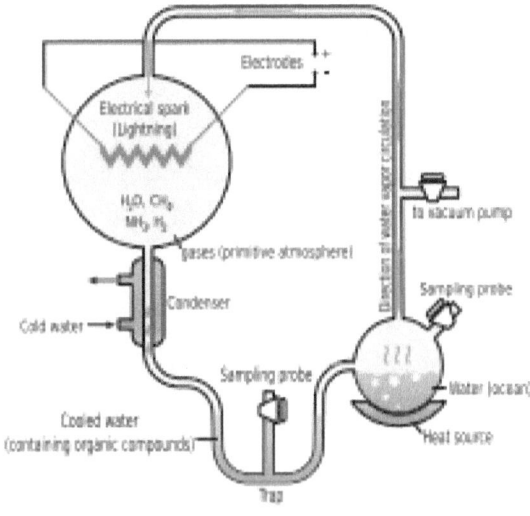

Fig. 5.2

- *The 1934 Nobel Prize in Chemistry was awarded to Harold Clayton Urey "for his discovery of heavy hydrogen."... In 1953, he was part of the famous Miller-Urey experiment.*
  - [1934 Nobel Prize in Chemistry] nobelprize.org
- In 2020, a study of magma from about 4.5 billion years ago suggested that Earth's original atmosphere contained little oxygen and no methane or ammonia, as assumed in the Miller-Urey experiment.
  - [magma] [Miller-Urey experiment] wikipedia
    - A study by researcher Dr. Tanai Cardona showed that a primitive form of photosynthesis that did not generate oxygen evolved in bacteria more than 3.5 billion years ago.
      - [no oxygen photosynthesis] sciencedaily
        - Cyanobacteria have the oldest known fossils, about 3.5 billion years old.
          - [record fossil cyanobacteria] berkeley.edu

- ⊕ Then, about 500 million years later, a new form of photosynthesis that generated oxygen emerged, called oxygenic photosynthesis.
  - [oxygenic photosynthesis] wikipedia
  - ⊕ Under certain conditions, when CO2 and H2O are exposed to sunlight, a chemical reaction occurs, which we can summarize with the following expression:
    - ⊕ CO2 + H2O + *photons* => *carbohidrates* + O2.
      - [photons] [carbohydrates] wikipedia
    - ⊕ Photons are elementary particles with no mass and are the basic units of light.
    - ⊕ Carbohydrates (made from C, H, and O) will be a fundamental block in creating the biomolecules ATP, RNA, and DNA, described later.
      - [carbohydrates] [ATP] [RNA] [DNA] wikipedia
      - *The 1970 Nobel Prize in Chemistry was awarded to Luis Leloir "for his discovery of sugar nucleotides and their role in carbohydrate biosynthesis."*
        - [1970 Nobel Prize in Chemistry]] nobelprize.org
  - ⊕ Note: Oxygenic photosynthesis is considered Earth's most crucial evolutionary innovation.
    [evolutionary innovation] news.mit.edu
  - ⊕ Oxygenic photosynthesis will be the process by which cyanobacteria, algae, and plants will use the sun's energy to produce sugar and release oxygen, as shown in the following figure.
    - [cyanobacteria] [photosynthesis] wikipedia

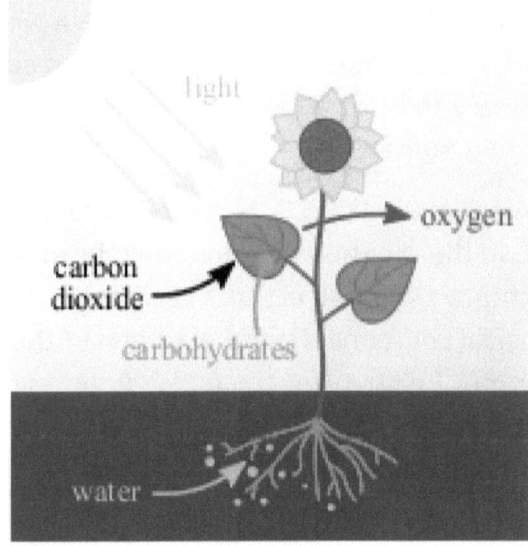

Fig. 5.3

- ◉ Note: The origin and evolution of photosynthesis are considered the key to the origin of life.
  - [photosynthesis and the origin of life] pubmed [Purple Earth hypothesis]
- ◉ Note: ATP (adenosine triphosphate) will be our most important source of mechanical and chemical energy. The chapter 'ATP Batteries' covers ATP in more detail.
  - ◉ The ATP hypothesis explains the central role of ATP in the origin of genetic codes and how this would be the key to revealing the origin of life on Earth since it is a prerequisite for its existence.
    - [ATP hypothesis] pdf
- ◉ Then biopolymers emerge. They are macromolecules composed of many repeated subunits called monomers. They form structured chains to construct important biological components, such as lipids, nucleotides, nucleic acids like RNA, DNA, and amino acids.
  - [biopolymers] [monomers] [biomolecular structure] wikipedia

- ○ ⊕ Note: We will see how RNA and DNA will be used as lasting information storage centers to store the code necessary to build all kinds of biological robots, including humans.

1. ⊕ Lipids (made from C, H, and O) are the fundamental block in the creation of bilipid membranes. These membranes form structures used to encapsulate/isolate biological components and play one of the most important functions in the development of life and human beings.
   - [lipidos] [membranas bilípidas] [membranas biológicas] wikipedia

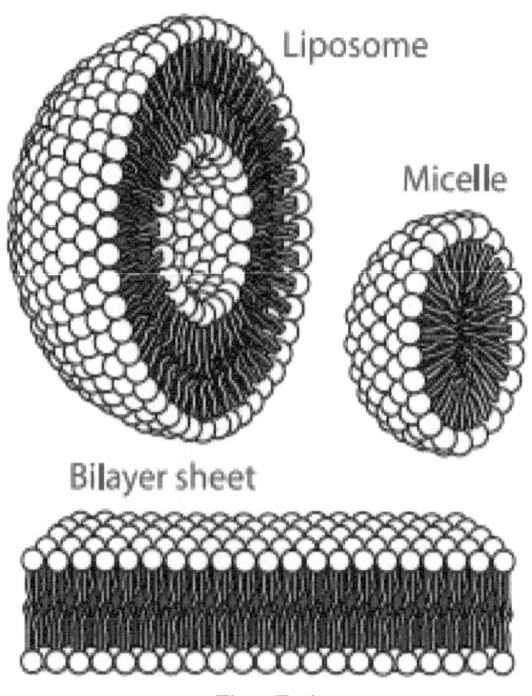

Fig. 5.4

   - ⊕ The figure above shows the different types of structures that can be formed with membranes made of lipids.

- ◈ Bilipid membranes can self-assemble and close into small vesicles (bio-containers), as shown in the following figure.
  - [vesicles] wikipedia

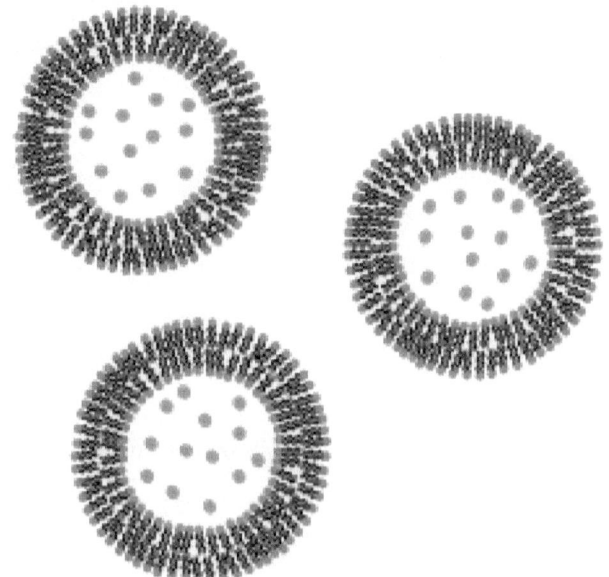

Fig. 5.5

- ◈ The vesicles will be used as isolation chambers for chemical reactions. They form compartments that are separated from the external environment, thus providing specialized functionality in a) aqueous spaces in temporary storage, b) transporting food and biochemical components, c) in buoyancy control, and more.

  - *The 2013 Nobel Prize in Physiology or Medicine was jointly awarded to James E. Rothman, Randy W. Schekman, and Thomas C. Sudhof "for their discoveries of the machinery that regulates vesicle trafficking, an important transport system in our cells."*
    - [2013 Nobel Prize in Physiology or Medicine] nobelprize.org

- ⊕ The cell membranes of almost all organisms and many viruses are bilipid membranes.
- ⊕ The following video by Jack Szostak (Harvard/HHMI) explains protocellular membranes.
  - [Part 2: Protocell Membranes] youtube

2. ⊕ Nucleotides: Here, we will explore RNA nucleotides and DNA nucleotides.
   - [RNA] [DNA] wikipedia

   - ⊕ RNA nucleotides are the structural blocks of RNA. Each is made up of a phosphate that binds the nucleotides together and a sugar that binds the nucleobase. The figure shows a simplified model of a single chain of RNA nucleotides.
     - [ribonucleotide] wikipedia

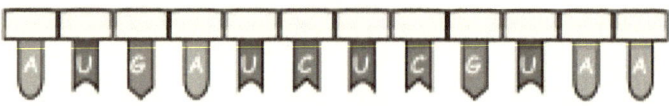

Fig. 5.6

   - ⊕ The nucleobases can only be A(adenine), G(guanine), C(cytosine), and U(uracil), and the combinations of these will be part of the genetic code.
     - [nucleobases] [genetic code] wikipedia

   - ⊕ According to complementarity, the nucleobases of the RNA only pair with their complements, as indicated in the figure.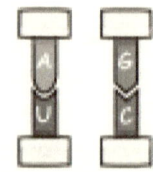
     - [complementarity] wikipedia

- ⊕ DNA nucleotides are the structural blocks of DNA; each is made up of a phosphate that binds the

nucleotides together and a sugar that binds the nucleobase. The following figure shows a simplified model of a single chain of DNA nucleotides.

- [polynucleotide]] [DNA nucleotides]

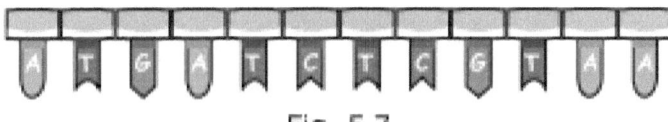

Fig. 5.7

- ◈ The nucleobases can only be A(adenine), G(guanine), C(cytosine), and T(thymine), and the combinations of these will be part of the genetic code.
  - [nucleobases] [nucleobases] wikipedia

- ◈ The T in DNA is distinguished from the U in RNA and has been considered an evolutionary change that strengthened DNA.

- ◈ According to complementarity, DNA nucleobases only pair with their complements, as indicated in the figure on the right.

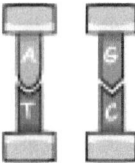

- ◈ The following figure shows an example of a double strand of DNA nucleotides made of two complementary single chains.
  - [DNA nucleotide] wikipedia

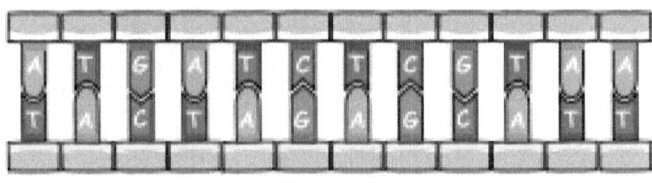

Fig. 5.8

- ◈ Since the principle of complementarity governs nucleobases, the chains of RNA and DNA nucleotides can be easily replicated and repaired.

- [complementarity] wikipedia

---

3. ⊕ The nucleic acids RNA and DNA are formed by chains of nucleotides RNA and DNA, respectively, and these are nothing less than the most important biomolecular components of living beings.

    - ⊕ *The 1959 Nobel Prize in Physiology or Medicine was awarded jointly to Severo Ochoa and Arthur Kornberg "for their discovery of the mechanisms in the biological synthesis of ribonucleic acid and deoxyribonucleic acid"... Ochoa and Marianne Grunberg-Manago discovered an enzyme in 1955 that can join nucleotides.*
        - [1959 Nobel Prize in Physiology or Medicine] nobelprize.org

    - ⊕ The following figure shows the structures of RNA, DNA, and their corresponding nucleobases:
        - [Difference DNA RNA] wikimedia

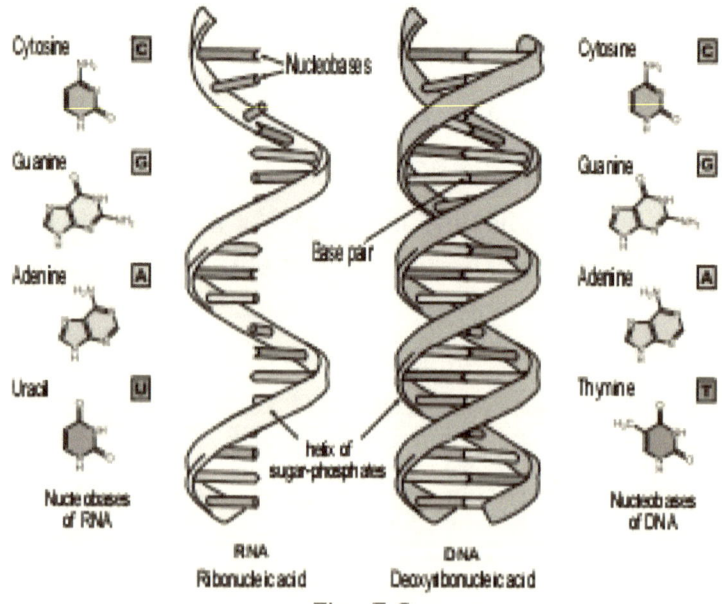

Fig. 5.9

> - *The 1910 Nobel Prize in Physiology or Medicine was awarded to Albrecht Kossel "in recognition of contributions to our knowledge of cellular chemistry through his work on proteins, including nucleic substances."*
>   - *[1910 Nobel Prize in Physiology or Medicine] nobelprize.org*

4. ⊕ Proteinogenic amino acids are a group of 22 amino acids that play a very important role in synthesizing peptides and proteins.
   - [proteinogenic amino acids] [peptides] [proteins] wikipedia

- ⊕ The nucleic acids RNA and DNA will be used as lasting information storage centers. The more stable DNA, which offers greater capacity, will be used to store all the information necessary to build a human being.

- ⊕ Note: The carbohydrates, proteins, lipids, and nucleic acids will allow life to exist.

- ⊕ Note: Vital matter is used to create all known life forms and comes in three forms: RNA, DNA, and proteins.

- ⊕ The first molecular robots emerge through a natural process from RNA nucleotide sequences, giving rise to the ring of the mind of molecular robots.

eduardo padilla-diaz

Rings-3

① *"Explores from the minds of molecular robots to the origins of life."*

6.1 Introduction

- ◉ Reflections on the rings of the mind (part 3):
- ①◉ As we saw in the previous chapter, the molecular mind gave rise to the existence of the mind of molecular robots, which is described below:

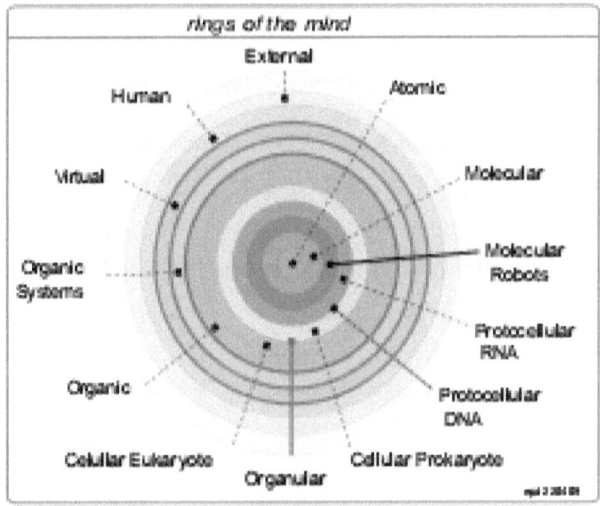

Fig. 6.1

6.2 Mind of the Molecular Robots

- ◉ The mind of molecular robots governs their minds and behaviors. Molecular robots are made of vital matter, initially RNA, but as we will see, they will become encoded in DNA through evolution. They are in charge of carrying out very useful vital functions. Each molecular robot's intelligence, operability, functionality, and morphology vary according to the nucleotide sequences used to create it.

- 🌑 Molecular robots will give rise to two important vital beings: ribozymes and viroids.
  ◦ [ribozymes] [viroids] wikipedia

1. ⊕ Ribozymes are molecular robots with great intelligence. They can create the set of chemical reactions that sustain an organism's life (metabolism); they self-catalyze (accelerate) their chemical reactions, self-replicate, and synthesize other types of RNA molecules. With all this, they make the existence of life.
    - [ribozymes] wikipedia [ribozymes] chemistry world

    - ⊕ A catalyst is a substance that accelerates the speed of a chemical reaction millions of times; reactions that take years can occur in fractions of seconds, as the figure shows.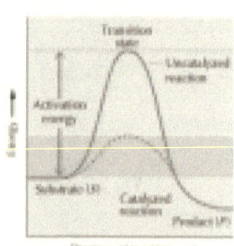
        - [catalysis] wikipedia

    - ⊕ The figure on the right shows a simplified model of a ribozyme. The YouTube video "RNA world hypothesis" is an 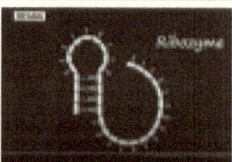 excellent exposition of how ribozymes could be formed.
        - [RNA world hypothesis by Stated Clearly] youtube

    - ⊕ In 1982, Thomas Cech and his team discovered an in vitro RNA sequence capable of cleaving itself without any protein or external energy source. Shortly after, Sid Altman's group demonstrated that

an RNA component could also be processed without protein. Cech and Altman shared the 1989 Nobel Prize in Chemistry for this work.
- [Ribozymes the characteristics and properties of catalytic RNAs] academic.oup.com

  - *The Nobel Prize in Chemistry - 1989, was awarded to Thomas R. Cech and Sidney Altman for their discovery of the catalytic properties of RNA. Ribozymes were first discovered in Cech's laboratory in 1982.*
    - [1989 Nobel Prize in Chemistry] nobelprize.org

2. ⊕ Viroids are infectious agents that cause infection in the susceptible host, like viruses. They are made up of a short cyclic chain of RNA. They appear as naked RNA; they do not have coverage. They constitute a primitive stage of viruses.
   - [viroids] [viroid] wikipedia

     - ⊕ The figure below shows the assembly schematic of the potato viroid ("PSTVd"), the first viroid to be identified. It is a small single-stranded circular RNA molecule of 359 nucleotides.
       - [potato viroid] wikipedia

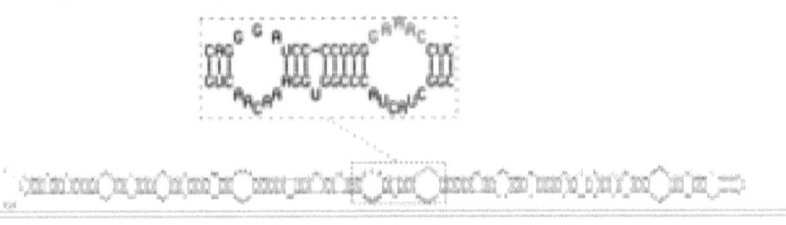

- ⊕ The significance of the evolution of RNA molecular robots will be such that it will lead, in later rings, to the creation of more than 1,300 types of molecular robots made of proteins, which will be much more intelligent and sophisticated, which will be key in the construction of cells and will be discussed later.

- ⊕ The evolution of RNA molecular robots will give rise to the ring of the protocellular mind.

6.3 RNA protocellular mind

- ⊕ The RNA protocellular mind governs the RNA protocells, the most primitive cells that fulfill the minimum vital functions necessary to give rise to the origins of life.

- ⊕ The figure shows what may have been an RNA protocell, consisting mainly of a protection and insulation capsule (bilipid membrane); several strands of RNA, which contain the genome; ribozymes; and other components necessary in the conversion of food into fuel, and in its self-replication.

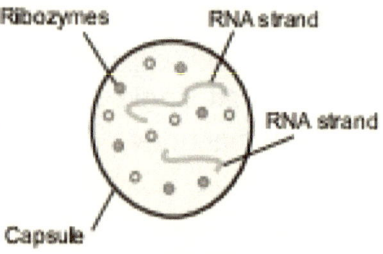

Fig. 6.2

- ⊕ There are several hypotheses about the origins of life, but here, we will only consider the RNA World, the Ganti Chemothon, and the RNP World.

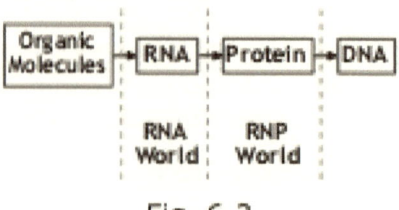

Fig. 6.3

1. ◉ The RNA World hypothesis, proposed by Alexander Rich in 1962, establishes a hypothetical stage in the evolutionary history of proteins and explains how these molecules could be formed:
   - [RNA World] [Alexander Rich] wikipedia

   - ◉ Researchers at Simon Fraser University produced random RNA sequences and surprisingly proved that nucleotides could be produced. Successful sequences were selected, and then, using a PCR technique, they were replicated with slight random mutations. After only 10 rounds of PCR, followed by selection, highly efficient nucleotide-building ribozymes were obtained (evolved) and exhibited the ability to participate actively in their own survival!
     - [Simón Fraser University] wikipedia [PCR] nature

     - *The 1993 Nobel Prize in Chemistry was awarded "for contributions to the development of methods within DNA-based chemistry," half to Kary B. Mullis "for her invention of the PCR method," and half to Michael Smith "for his fundamental contributions to the establishment of oligonucleotide-based site-directed mutagenesis and its development for protein studies."*
       - [1993 Nobel Prize in Chemistry] nobelprize.org

   - ◉ Ribozymes, together with viroids, currently constitute the only RNA molecules that support this theory and probably those that have participated in the abiogenesis process.
     - [abiogenesis] [viroids] wikipedia

2. ◉ Ganti's Chemothon:

   - ◉ In 1952, Tibor Gánti introduced an abstract model for the fundamental unit of life that he called the Chemoton (chemical automaton). In 1971, he formulated the concept in his book "The Principles of

Life." He suggested that the Chemoton was the original ancestor of all organisms.
- [chemoton] [tibor ganti] wikipedia
  - ⊕ The Chemoton model establishes that life must have three fundamental properties: metabolism, self-replication, and a bilipid membrane.
    - [metabolism] [bilipid membranes] wikipedia
3. ⊕ The RNP world is a hypothetical intermediate period in the origin of life characterized by the existence of proteins. The period followed the hypothetical RNA world and ended with the formation of DNA and contemporary proteins, which led to life as we know it.
   - [RNP world] wikipedia

- ⊕ In 1950, Renato Dulbecco discovered that certain viruses work by incorporating their DNA into the DNA of host cells. In 1970, David Baltimore and Howard Temin, independently of each other, discovered that viruses with RNA genomes can also insert themselves into the DNA of host cells. The discovery that information from RNA can be transferred to DNA (reverse transcription) meant that the generally accepted rule that genetic information is only transferred in one direction: DNA to RNA, RNA to protein, had to be modified.
  - [RT reverse transcribed] pubmed.ncbi.nlm.nih.gov

    - ⊕ *The 1975 Nobel Prize in Physiology or Medicine was awarded jointly to David Baltimore, Renato Dulbecco, and Howard Martin Temin "for their discoveries on the interaction between tumor viruses and the genetic material of the cell."*
      - [1975 Nobel Prize in Physiology/Medicine] nobelprize.org
    - ⊕ The central dogma of molecular biology explains the flow of genetic information within a biological system.

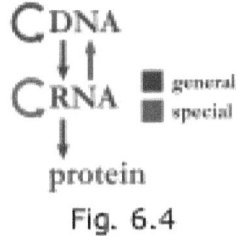

Fig. 6.4

- The figure shows the flow of genetic information, from which we can infer two types of transfers:

  - ◈ General transfers: DNA can be copied (replication); DNA information can be transcribed into an RNA template (transcription); and RNA templates are used to synthesize proteins (translation).

  - ◈ The special transfers are that RNA can be copied (replication), and information from RNA can be transcribed and inserted into DNA (reverse transcription).

- ◈ The evolution of the RNP world will lead to the supremacy of DNA and contemporary proteins. By then, the laws governing how all essential gene products in all life forms are encoded, stored, extracted, and synthesized will be well defined.

- ◈ The evolution of the RNA protocellular mind ring will give rise to the DNA protocellular mind ring.

6.4 DNA Protocellular Mind

- ◈ The DNA protocellular mind governs the DNA protocells, the most primitive cells that fulfill the minimum vital functions necessary to give rise to the origins of life.

- ⊕ The figure shows what may have been a DNA protocell. It consists mainly of a protective and isolating capsule (bilipid membrane), the protocellular genome, ribozymes, and other active components that we will see below.
  - [Prokaryotic Cell Diagram] wikipedia

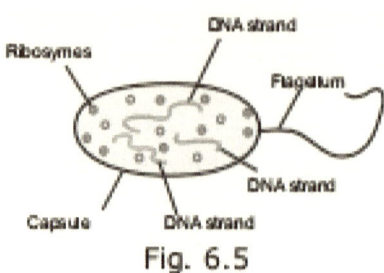

Fig. 6.5

- ⊕ The protocellular genome contains, in a chain of DNA nucleotides, all the information necessary to create all the components that a proto-cell needs for it to operate and function correctly, including ribozymes, mRNA, tRNA-ligase, tRNA, ribosomes, proteins, and enzymes. These components will also be used in the different types of cells appearing in the next rings of the mind.
  1. ⊕ The ribozymes are molecular robots, which we covered in the previous section.
  2. ⊕ The mRNA (template) represents the genetic schematic of a gene component. When the gene for a protein is extracted from the genome, it is extracted into an mRNA template that a ribosome molecular robot can read to synthesize.
     - [mRNA] [gene] [ribosoma] wikipedia
  3. ⊕ Ribosomes are molecular robots that synthesize proteins by reading mRNA templates. A template can represent anything from a small chain of amino acids or peptides to a large chain that forms a protein.
     - [ribosome] wikipedia

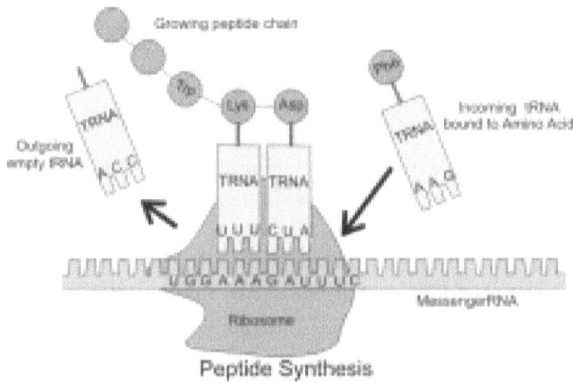

Peptide Synthesis
Fig. 6.6

- ☯ The figure illustrates how the ribosome, assisted by multiple tRNAs and other components, selects amino acids and assembles a protein according to an mRNA template.

- *The Nobel Prize in Chemistry - 2009 was awarded to Venkatraman Ramakrishnan, Thomas A. Steitz, and Ada E. Yonath "for their studies on the structure and function of the ribosome."*
  - [2009 Nobel Prize in Chemistry] nobelprize.org

4. ☯ tRNA-ligase is a molecular robot that loads the appropriate amino acid into a corresponding tRNA.
   - [tRNA] wikipedia [tRNA-ligase] wikipedia

5. ☯ The tRNA is a molecular robot that delivers an amino acid to a protein synthesizer ribosome.
   - [tRNA] wikipedia [tRNA-ligase] wikipedia

6. ☯ Proteins are made up of one or more chains of protein amino acids. They are the third version of vital matter, which is much more complete and stable. They are divided into several branches, but we will only cover enzymes for now.

   - ☯ Enzymes: They are molecular robots that perform a wide variety of functions, such as catalysts and motors.

- ⊕ Catalysts are chemical molecular robots that accelerate chemical reactions, such as orotidine, which accelerates a reaction to milliseconds that would otherwise take millions of years.
  - [enzyme] wikipedia [enzymes as catalysts] ncbi.nlm.nih.gov
- ⊕ Motors: such as the flagellum, which is a molecular rotation motor used to propel certain cells. The following video by Michael Behe shows the amazing flagellum motor.
  - [Amazing Flagellum : Michael Behe and the Revolution of Intelligent Design] youtube

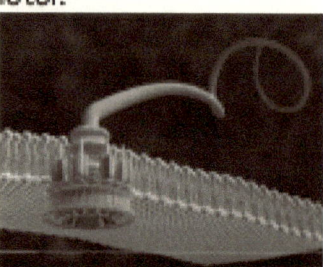

- ⊕ The evolution of DNA protocells will give rise to the ring of the prokaryotic cellular mind.

6.5 Prokaryotic Cellular Mind

- ⊕ The prokaryotic cellular mind is that which governs all bacteria and archaea. They are powerful cellular robots governed by bio-operating systems. They are unicellular organisms that lack a nucleus. Their morphology and purpose vary depending on how the genes that form them are expressed. Their genomes include all the information necessary to build them and allow them to grow and reproduce; they can move to find food or escape predators; some have motor flagella and cilia to mobilize; they form a biomass that exceeds all plants and animals. Later, we will see that the eukaryotic cells that make up our body descend from prokaryotic cells.

- [prokaryote] [origin of the first cell] wikipedia [bio-operating systems] [universal ancestor] pnas.org

- ⊙ Our body depends on bacteria to survive since only they can synthesize the vitamin B12 necessary in metabolism; some are pathogenic and cause infectious diseases. The figure shows the typical structure of a bacteria (0.2-2um).
  - [bacteria] wikipedia

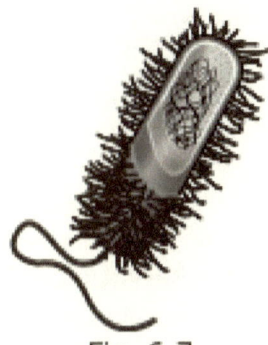

Fig. 6.7

- ⊙ The following figure shows a T4 bacteriophage virus (~90nm) that infects a certain type of bacteria, resulting in the total destruction of the infected bacteria. Image courtesy of Víctor Padilla-Sánchez, PhD.
  - [bacteriophage T4] wikipedia

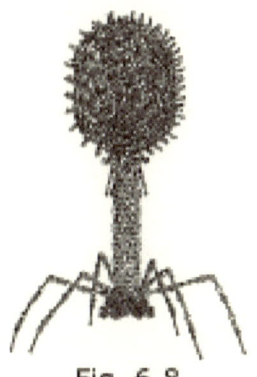

Fig. 6.8

- ◉ The following figure shows the typical structure of archaea (1-1.5um). Archaea are very similar to bacteria, but their genomes are very different.
  - [archaea] rsscience.com

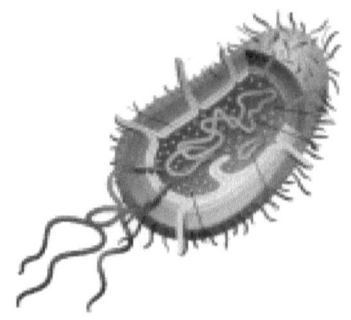

Fig. 6.9

- ◉ The evolution of prokaryotic cells will give rise to the ring of the eukaryotic cellular mind.

- ◉ The illustration shows the phylogenetic tree of life.
  - [phylogenetic tree] wikipedia

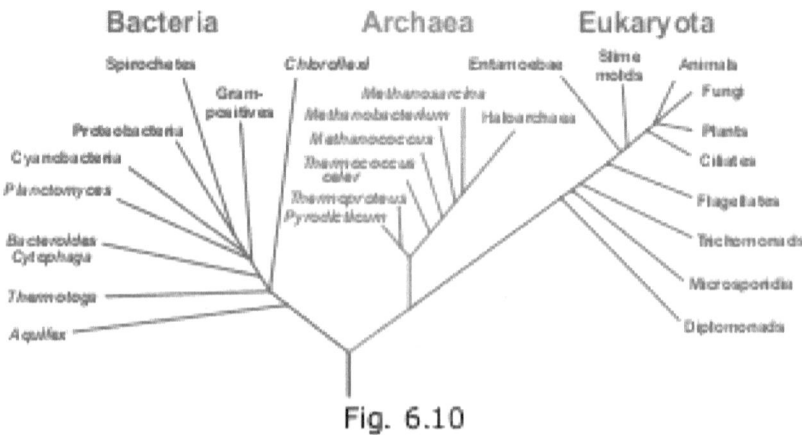

Fig. 6.10

- ◉ The endosymbiotic theory states that eukaryotes arose as a result of a fusion of archaean with bacteria, where an ancient archaean engulfed (but did not eat) an ancient aerobic bacteria; it remained within the archaea in what

may have been a mutualistic relationship: the engulfed bacteria allowed the host archaea to use oxygen to release energy stored in nutrients, and the host archaea protected the bacteria from predators. Over many generations, a symbiotic relationship developed between the two organisms so complete that neither could survive on its own. Microfossil evidence suggests that eukaryotes emerged sometime between 1.6 billion to 2.2 billion years ago. The descendants of this ancient engulfing cell are present in all eukaryotic cells today as mitochondria.
  - [eukaryotes-and-their-origins] gatech.edu

6.6 Organular Mind

- 🔹 The organular mind is the mind that governs each of the small organs, called organelles, that can become part of each cell. Each organelle is a powerful robot with great intelligence; its morphology, operability, and functionality vary according to the genes that are activated to create it.
  - [organel] [serial endosymbiosis.svg] wikipedia [serial endosymbiosis.svg] wikimedia

    - 🔹 Organular robots are protected by their own bio-packaging.

    - 🔹 Prokaryotic cells only consist of an organelle robot, while eukaryotic cells have several types.

    - 🔹 Within eukaryotic cells, we can find the following organular robots: nucleus, mitochondria, endoplasmic reticulum, lysosome, Golgi apparatus, centrosome, and vacuole.
      - [organel] [nucleus] [nucleus] [[endoplasmic reticulum] [[lysosome] [golgi apparatus] [centrosome] [vacuole] wikipedia

- ◈ To give us an idea of the complexity and level of intelligence of these organelles, for now, we are only going to cover the following: the mitochondria and the Golgi apparatus:

    - ◈ The mitochondria (1um: ~50-2000) are semi-autonomous organular robots found in most eukaryotic cells. Their number per cell can vary widely; for example, red blood cells nuke their nuclei and have no mitochondria, while liver cells can have more than 2000. Mitochondria have their own DNA; they self-replicate and supply cellular energy ATP. They participate in other tasks, such as signaling, cell differentiation, and cell death.
        - [mitochondria] [mitochondrial DNA] [ATP] wikipedia [red blood cells nuke their nuclei] wi.mit.edu

    - ◈ The figure shows the structure of a mitochondrion.

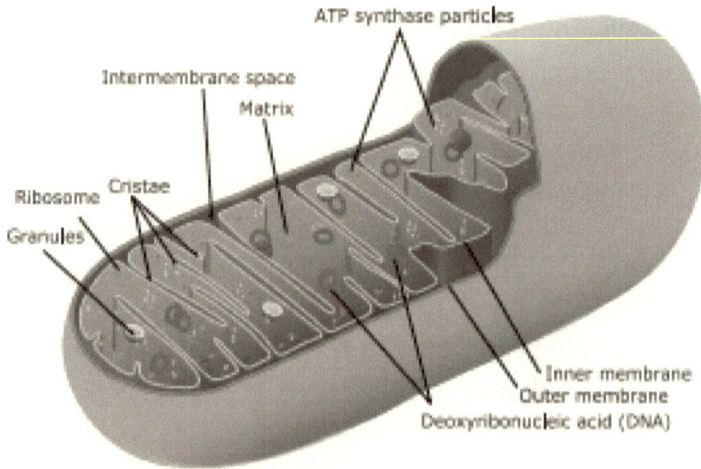

Fig. 6.11

    - ◈ Human mitochondrial DNA was the first significant part of the human genome to be sequenced, and it revealed that it includes 16,569 base pairs and encodes 13 proteins.

- ◈ The Golgi apparatus (2um: 1) is an organelle robot that functions as a post office. It performs the following: a) receives proteins manufactured by ribosomes; b) packs them in protective envelopes; c) labels them; d) sends them to one of four possible destinations: cell plasma, cell membrane, outside the cell, or the waste center.
  - ◈ The figure shows the structure of the Golgi apparatus.

Fig. 6.12

- *The 1999 Nobel Prize in Physiology or Medicine was awarded to Gunter Blobel "for the discovery that proteins have intrinsic signals that govern their transport and localization in the cell."*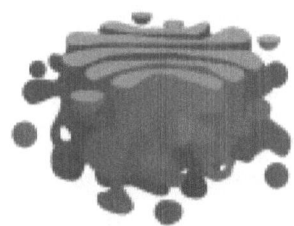
  - [1999 Nobel Prize in Physiology or Medicine] nobelprize.org

6.7 Eukaryotic Cellular Mind

- ◈ The eukaryotic cellular mind is the mind that governs each of the cells that the human body has. It is estimated that the human body has around 37 trillion cells. Each cell is a powerful robot - which we will call a cellular robot - that has great intelligence and can perform useful and highly complex vital functions. There

are two main types of cells: somatic cells and reproductive cells.
- [cell] wikipedia

- ⊚ Somatic cells: The human body has more than 200 different types of these cells, such as neurons, epithelial cells, and leukocytes, which are found in the nervous system, skin, and blood, respectively. However, although somatic cells are very diverse in their form and function, they are all identical genetically because they do not express all their genes but only those of the cell group to which they belong. This process is called cellular differentiation, which occurs from the embryonic stage. Thus, certain genes are active in some cells and inactive in others. Because somatic cells do not participate in sexual reproduction, mutations can affect the individual but are not transmitted to their offspring.

  - The figure shows the structure of a typical somatic cell.

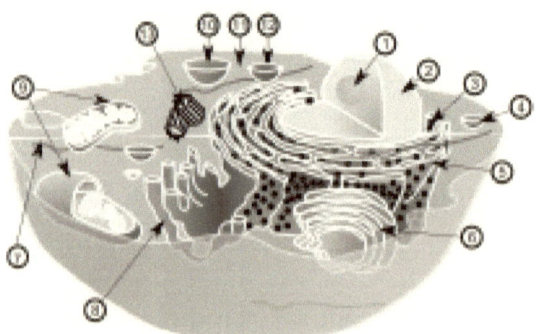

Fig. 6.13

1 nucleolus, 2 nucleus, 3 ribosome, 4 vesicles, 5 rough reticulum, 6 golgi apparatus, 7 cytoskeleton, 8 smooth reticulum, 9 mitochondria, 10 vacuole, 11 cytosol, 12 lysosome, 13 centriole.

- *The 1974 Nobel Prize in Physiology or Medicine was awarded jointly to Albert Claude, Christian de Duve, and George E. Palade "for their discoveries on the structural and functional organization of the cell."*
  - [1974 Nobel Prize in Physiology or Medicine] nobelprize.org
- The figure shows the typical membrane structure that encloses a cell.
  - [membrane] wikipedia

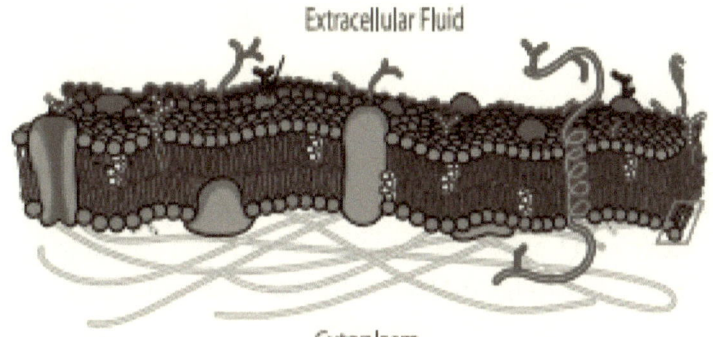

Fig. 6.14

- Reproductive cells: They are made up of eggs and sperm and are used to create new human beings through fertilization. The chapter Life explores this topic in greater detail.

6.8 Organic Mind

- The organic mind is the mind that governs each of the organs of the human body. The human body has about 100 different types of organs, including the brain, heart, lungs, liver, kidneys, bladder, stomach, intestines, eyes, ears, bones, muscles, and many more. Here, we will not detail the specific functionality of each organ. What interests us in the context of this exploration is to know that each organ is a powerful organic robot - that

has great intelligence and performs important functions for one or several organic systems, such as, for example, the lungs that work for the respiratory system.
    - [[organic systems] [organs of the human body] wikipedia
- 🕐🔶 The organic mind and its inner rings give rise to the existence of the mind of organic systems.

6.9 Mind of Organic Systems

- 🕐🔶 The minds of the organic systems govern the minds of the following systems: musculoskeletal, nervous, motor, digestive, respiratory, urinary, reproductive, endocrine (hormones), blood, lymphatic (defense), sensory (visual, auditory, olfactory, gustatory), somatosensory (touch, temperature, body position, pain), integumentary (skin, hair, nails), and others. Here, we are not going to go into detail about the specific functionality of each of them. What interests us in the context of this exploration is knowing that each of these is composed of several organic robots, several types of tissues, and various kinds of fluids, which together form a giant robot of great intelligence that performs important functions for one or several organic systems.
    - [organic systems] [organs of the human body] [digestive system] wikipedia

- As an example of the complexity of an organic system, the figure shows the digestive system:

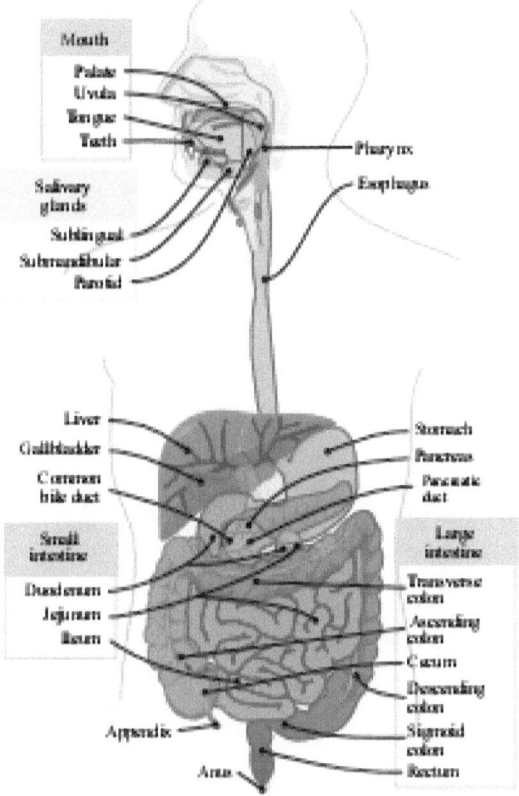

Fig. 6.15

- ↑● The minds of the organic systems and their inner rings give rise to the existence of the virtual mind.

eduardo padilla-diaz

Rings-4

❶ *"Explores from the virtual mind to the human and external minds."*

7.1 Introduction

- ◆ Reflections on the rings of the mind (part 4):
- ❶◆ As we saw in the previous chapter, the minds of organic systems and their inner rings give rise to the existence of the virtual mind.

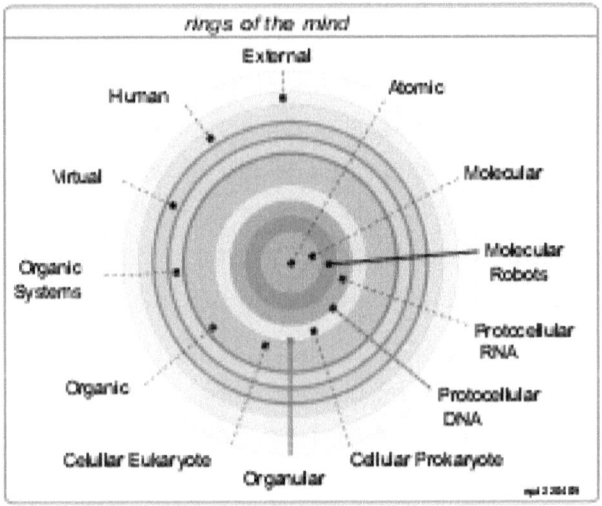

Fig. 7.1

7.2 Virtual Mind

- ❶◆ The virtual mind is the mind that governs the virtual organs, which are nothing more than processors located mainly in the brain, made by billions of neurons assisted by billions of glial cells. Virtual organs perform unique

and highly sophisticated functions, such as imagination, thinking, attention, understanding, comprehension, intelligence, awareness, consciousness, reason, etc. These virtual organs are the fundamental basis of the human mind and are explored throughout this adventure. Its architecture is very complex, and so is its interconnectivity; it requires several stops on this adventure to describe and model them in detail.
    - [brain] [neurons] [glial cells] wikipedia
- ◐ The virtual mind and its inner rings give rise to the existence of the human mind.

7.3 Human Mind

- ◐ The human mind is in charge of the operation and functionality of the largest of our biological robots: the human body. It includes the functionalities of all the other minds below this ring. It comprises the operational human mind and the functional human mind.
    - [mind] wikipedia
    - ◐ The operational human mind, which now includes virtual organs like attention, conscience, subconscience, thinking, and imagination, is responsible for our body's appropriate functioning in our physical environment. This mind is adaptive and evolves through learning and the expansion of acquired operational knowledge, thanks to the appearance of the subconscience and the semi-biobots. The subconscience and the semi-biobots are described later in other chapters.
        - ◆ Piaget's theory of cognitive development is still relevant and used in psychology. It maintains that the

construction of each human being is a process that occurs during the development of a person in childhood. The process is divided into four phases:
- [Piaget's theory of cognitive development] wikipedia

    1. ◆ Sensory-motor (0-2 years): The child uses his senses (fully developed) and motor skills to know what surrounds him.
    2. ◆ Preoperative (2-7 years): It is characterized by the internalization of the reactions of the previous phase, giving rise to mental actions that still need to be categorized as operations due to their vagueness, inadequacy, or lack of reversibility.
    3. ◆ Operational concrete (8-11 years) is the logical operations used to solve problems.
    4. ◆ Operational formal (12 years to adulthood): Intelligence is demonstrated through the logical use of symbols related to abstract concepts.

  o ◆◆ The functional human mind is the set of processes responsible for the joint functioning of our body, intellect, and emotions. It is adaptive and evolves through more advanced learning, resulting in better development of our physical, intellectual, emotional, and social faculties.

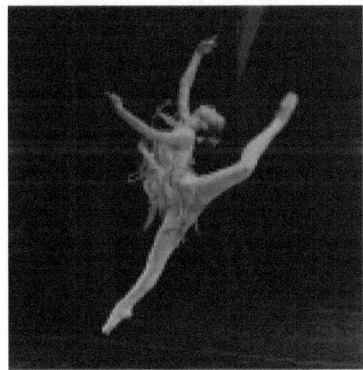

    - [Grace in winter, contemporary ballet] wikimedia

- ◆◆ The human mind and all its inner rings give rise to the existence of the external mind.

7.4 External Mind

- 🔹 The external mind is in charge of our body and the mind's interaction with other bodies, minds, and intelligent machines. There are many different types, and for now, we are going to limit them to unaware emotional, linguistic, moral, familial, marital, social, spiritual, and artificial:
    - 🔹 The unaware external emotional mind is responsible for unconsciously externalizing our emotional state to other beings and for us to capture unconsciously the emotional state of other beings.
    - 🔹 The linguistic external mind allows us to: a) communicate with other beings consciously; b) share stored knowledge with other beings; c) store and share knowledge in persistent media, such as books, audio and video recordings.
    - 🔹 The external moral mind ensures we behave appropriately with nature and other beings.
    - 🔹 The external familial mind is in charge of our interactions with family members' minds: to share experiences, learn what benefits us and what harms us, share what we learn, help and help us, and love and be loved.
    - 🔹 The conjugal external mind is responsible for interacting with the couple with whom we will preserve the species.
    - 🔹 The external social mind is responsible for helping us benefit from the knowledge of other minds in other bodies and their faculties. Thanks to the evolution of the external linguistic mind, we have created advanced

means of disseminating all types of knowledge through the Internet and social networks, allowing us to inform ourselves and share our experiences almost immediately in real-time.

- ◐◉ The external spiritual mind gives us a sense of where we came from before birth and where we go after death.
- ◐◉ The artificial external mind provides us with artificial physical and mental capabilities, such as artificial intelligence AI or augmented reality AR.
  - [AI - artificial intelligence] [AR - augmented reality] wikipedia

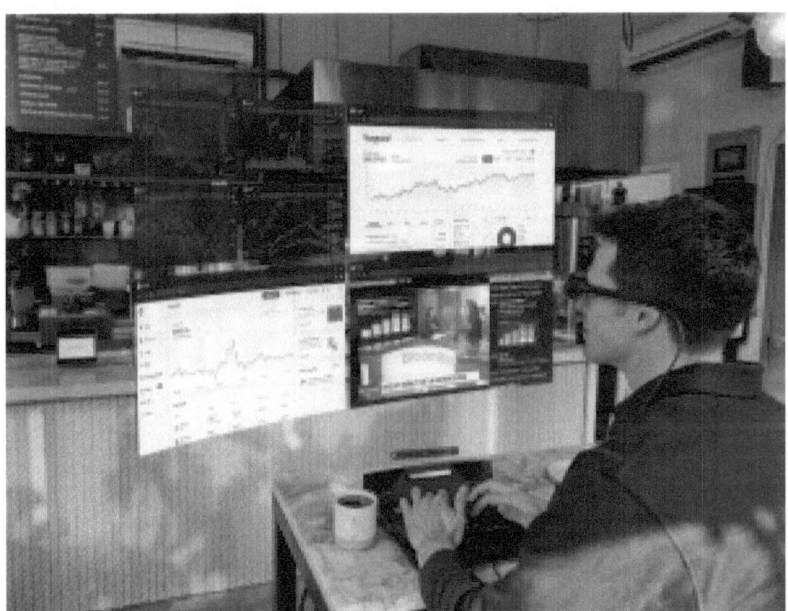

Fig. 7.2

- The photo shows how a person wearing AR Glasses can see a virtual multi-display system.
  - [Sightful-SPACETOP-G1] Sightful.com

- ◉ Note: It is important to note that the term mind will be used interchangeably in this book to refer to all the functions of all the minds stated in the last four chapters.

eduardo padilla-diaz

Vital Code

① *"Vital software is written with this code."*

8.1 Introduction

- ⊕ Reflections on the vital code:
- ⊕ First, let's explore certain informatics concepts: genetic code, human genome, genes, mRNA, and codons:
  1. ⊕ The genetic code uses combinations of four letters: A, G, C, and T to encode the informatic content in DNA and A, G, C, and U to encode the informatic content in RNA.
     - [genetic code] wikipedia

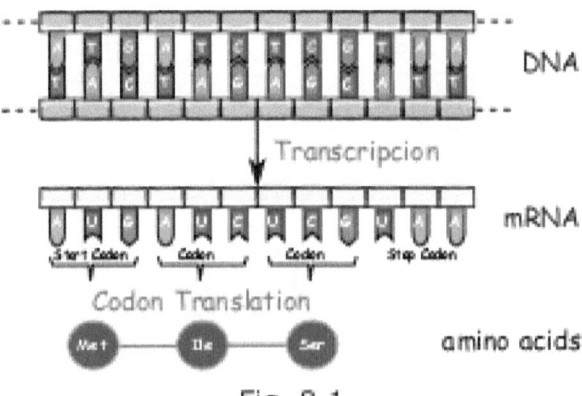

Fig. 8.1

  2. ⊕ The human genome contains the entire genetic code of a human being. It is made of DNA, found in the nucleus of every cell in the human body, and a tiny extension of the maternal genome is located in the mitochondria.
     - [human genome] wikipedia

3. ⊕ Genes are found in the genome and are sequences that encode gene products, such as the schematics of kinesin or dynein molecular robots.
    - [genes] wikipedia [kenesin and dynein molecular robots] sciencedirect.com
4. ⊕ The mRNA is a genetic template that represents a gene component. For example, the gene for a kinesin motor protein is extracted from the genome through transcription into an mRNA template. A ribosome molecular robot (see figure) reads the template using codon translation to build the kinesin motor as a sequence of amino acids.
    - [mRNA] [[transcription] [gene] [ribosome] [translation] wikipedia

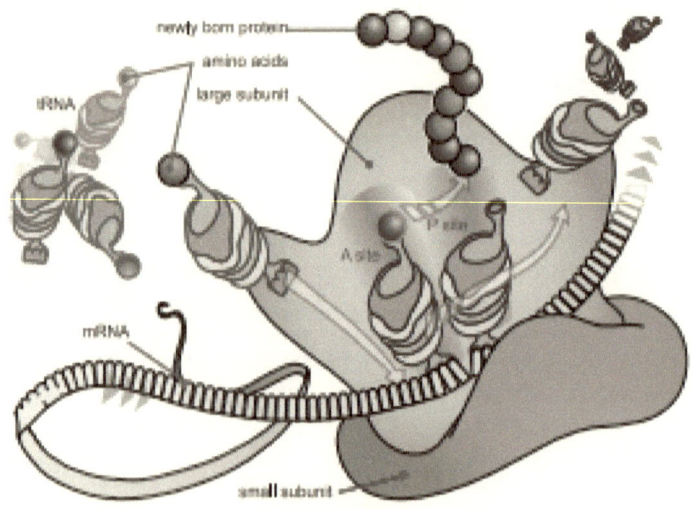

Fig. 8.2

5. ⊕ A codon is the triplet of RNA nucleotides (A, G, C, and U) used to form a specific amino acid. Codon sequences encode proteins through translation.
    - [proteinogenic amino acid]] [[translation] wikipedia [amino acid table] wikimedia

6. The following table shows the equivalence between codons and amino acids:

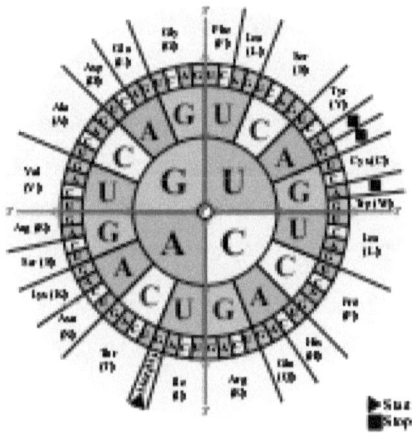

Fig. 8.3

- ◉ Example: the codon (AUG) represents the amino acid Met, a protein's start codon or first amino acid.
- ◉ Example: the codon (AUC) represents the amino acid Ile.
- ◉ Example: the (UAA) codon does not represent an amino acid but a stop codon that tells the protein synthesis machinery to terminate synthesis.

  - *The 1968 Nobel Prize in Physiology or Medicine was awarded jointly to Robert W. Holley, Har Gobind Khorana, and Marshall W. Nirenberg "for their interpretation of the genetic code and its role in protein synthesis."*
    - *[1968 Nobel Prize in Physiology or Medicine] nobelprize.org*

- ①◉ The vital code comprises DNA, RNA, or amino acid sequences.
  - [nucleotides] [RNA] [DNA] [amino acids] wikipedia

  1. ①◉ There are three types of vital code: passive, active and reactive:

a. 🔷 The passive vital code stores data, structures, and the schematics of vital beings. As we will see later, innate knowledge is stored in passive vital code.
b. 🔷 The active, vital code is used at the operational level in messages, data, and structures.
c. 🔷 The reactive vital code is used at a functional level to execute various molecular robot functions, such as accelerators of chemical reactions, mechanical workers, or reproducers of sensory excitations.
d. Generally, the term vital code can be applied to any of its types.

2. 🔷 There are two coding versions of the vital code: RNA and DNA-hybrid.
    a. 🔷 RNA coding is considered the oldest version, which is why it is attributed to the origin of life. Its passive, active, and reactive types use the same coding, based on combinations of four letters, A, G, C, and U, to encode the informatic content.
    b. 🔷 The DNA-hybrid coding is the second version, being much more complete, stable, and sophisticated. It allows for handling much more information than the RNA counterpart. Its passive type is based on DNA sequences arranged in complementary double strands, allowing the detection of assembly errors. The passive type is based on combinations of the four letters: A, G, C, and T. The active type is based on combinations of the four letters A, G, C, and U, and it is 100% compatible with the RNA active coding. The reactive type is based on combinations of 22 types of amino acids.

Memories-1

"Their physiology and where they are."

9.1 Introduction

- Reflections on memories (part 1):
- Memories are devices where information is stored to preserve it in an organized way so that it can be used in the future.
  - [memory] wikipedia
- Here, we will explore physiological memories to get an idea of the environment where they exist and what materials they are made of. These memories underlie all operational and functional memories, which we will discuss later.
  - [physiology] wikipedia
- Physiological memories are molecular devices where information is stored to preserve it in an organized way so that it can be used in the future. They are subdivided into DNA, mtDNA, and neuronal.

1. DNA memories are found in the nucleus of every cell in the body. Each cell stores a copy of the human genome (minus the extension of the maternal genome) in 6 billion base pairs of DNA. The human genome contains about 25,000 genes packed into several chromosomes.
   - [chromosomes] wikipedia [about red blood cells] [not all cells have the same DNA]
     a. The following figure shows how a typical cell contains a nucleus, how the nucleus stores

chromosomes, and how each chromosome stores part of the human genome in DNA.
  - [DNA] [chromosomes] wikipedia [Eukaryote DNA] wikimedia

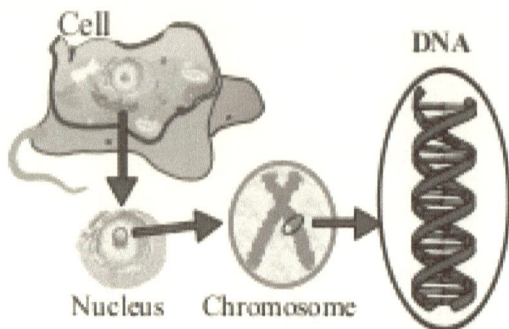

Fig. 9.1

b. ⊙ Each chromosome stores a different number of genes, which are the basic units of heredity and encode the synthesis of proteins, RNA, and other products. The following graph shows the distribution of our 25,000 genes on each of the chromosomes:
  - [gene] wikipedia [Genes and base pairs on chromosomes] wikimedia

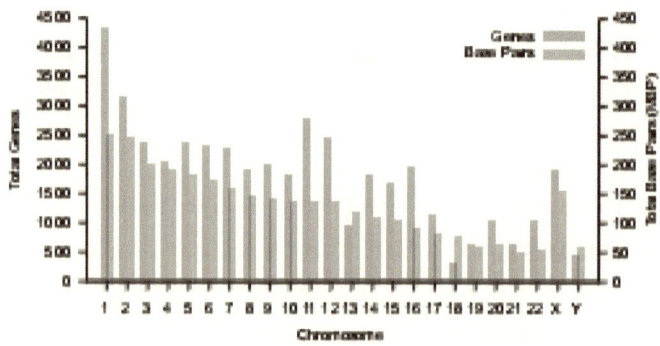

Fig. 9.2

c. ⊙ Of the 23 pairs of chromosomes, there are 22 pairs numbered from 1 to 22, where the mother and father contribute one chromosome of each pair to an offspring and a pair of sex chromosomes that

determine the sex of the offspring. The father can provide an X or a Y chromosome, while the mother always provides an X.
  - [human chromosomes] [facts about the Y chromosome] genome.gov

2. ◆ mtDNA memories are found in the mitochondria and different quantities in each cell. Each mitochondrion stores a copy of the maternal genome extension. The figure shows how, within a cell, mitochondria store several circular chromosomes, each with a complete copy of the length of the maternal genome:
   - [mtDNA] wikipedia [Mitochondrial DNA] wikimedia

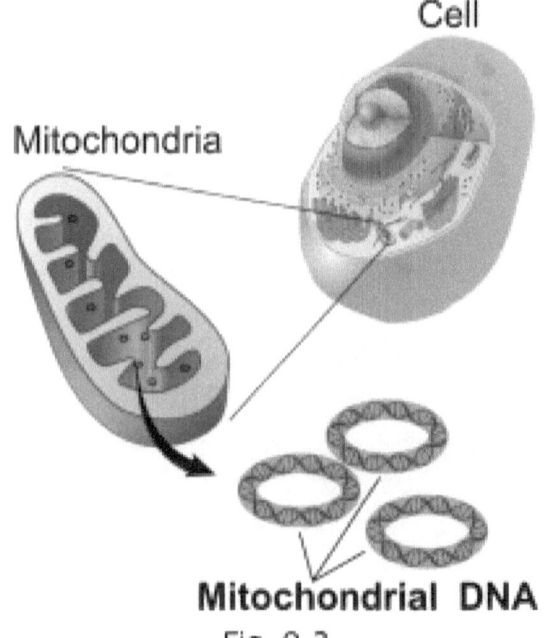

Fig. 9.3

a. ◆ The extension of the maternal genome is made by a circle of 16,569 base pairs of DNA containing 37 genes, which specify several molecular robots and several polypeptides.
   - [mtDNA] wikipedia

- ⊕ The following graphic, made by Emmanuel Douzery, shows the map of human mitochondrial genetics:
  - [mtDNA Map] [emmanuel douzery] wikipedia [Map of the human mitochondrial genome] wikimedia

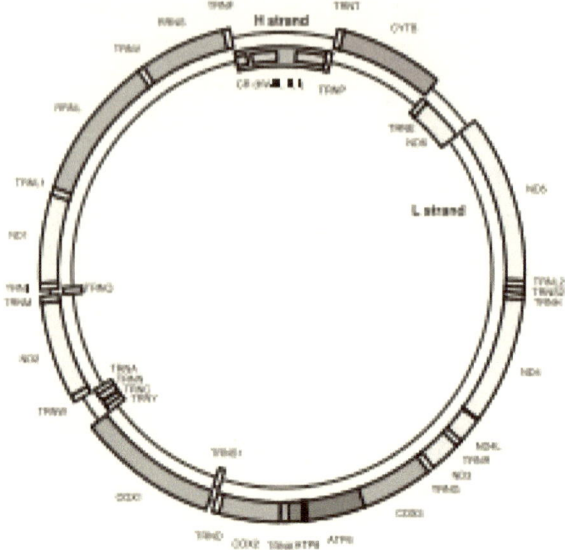

Fig. 9.4

- ⊕ One of the mtDNA genes contains the schematic of one of the most important molecular robots: the ATP synthase. This robot generates the ATP energy each cell needs to operate. The ATP Batteries chapter covers this molecular robot in more detail.
  - [ATP-synthase] wikipedia

3. ⊕ Neuronal memories: They are found within neurons and in their surroundings. Neurons interconnect with other neurons and cells, forming highly associative memory, control, and processing networks. It is estimated that the human body has around 86 billion neurons.

    The figure shows a typical neuron: it consists of a cell

body (soma), input connectors (dendrites), and a single axon where the output connectors (synapses) are located. Here, we are going to explore Intraneuronal memories and nECM memories:
- [neuronas] wikipedia [Complete neuron cell diagram] wikimedia

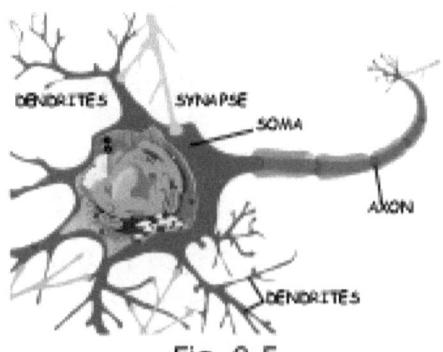

Fig. 9.5

a. ◆ Intraneuronal memories are found within neurons. The precise way in which information is encoded and stored within the memories of a neuron has not yet been able to be characterized. However, it is known that the number and strength of dendritic and synaptic connections are directly linked to our capacity for learning, memory, and cognition.

- ◆ Dendritic connections are the input connectors of a neuron made up of dendrites. They connect to synapses, which are the output connectors of other neurons.
  - [dendrite] wikipedia

  - ◆ In a single neuron, dendritic branching can be extensive and sufficient to receive up to 100,000 inputs.

  - ◆ Strength and quantity are related to learning, memory, and cognition.
    - [dentritic spines] Natural Library of Medicine

- ❖ Synaptic connections are the output connectors of a neuron; synapses form them. They allow a neuron to transmit signals to other neurons or other cells.
  - [synapse] wikipedia

- ❖ "Each synapse, in itself, is more like a microprocessor, with memory storage and information processing elements, than a simple on/off switch."
  - [brain connections] stanford medicine : stephen smith

- ❖ The number of synapses in a typical neuron varies between 1,000 to 10,000.
  - [brain figures] faculty.washington.edu

- ❖ The number of synapses in a Purkinje neuron (located in the cerebellum) is close to 200,000. The following figure illustrates this type, made by the Spaniard neuroscientist, pathologist, and histologist Santiago Ramón y Cajal, known as the father of modern neuroscience, Nobel 1906.
  - [purkinje neuron] [Santiago Ramón y Cajal] wikipedia [Cajal a purkinje neuron from the human cerebellum] wikimedia

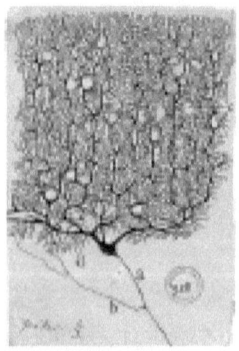

Fig. 9.6

- *The 1906 Nobel Prize in Physiology or Medicine was awarded jointly to Camillo Golgi and Santiago Ramón y Cajal " in recognition of their work on the structure of the nervous system ."*
  - [1906 Nobel Prize in Physiology or Medicine] nobelprize.org
- ◉ "In a human being, there are more than 125 trillion synapses in the cerebral cortex alone."
  - [conexiones cerebrales] stanford medicine : stephen smith

b. ◉ nECM memories are found around neurons within a neural extracellular matrix (nECM) network, which is much less prone to biodegradation. Compared to other types of memories, writing and reading in nECM memories are thousands of times faster, which aligns with the speed that short-term memories should have, where sensory information is stored in the process.
  - [nECM] interactive neuroscience journal

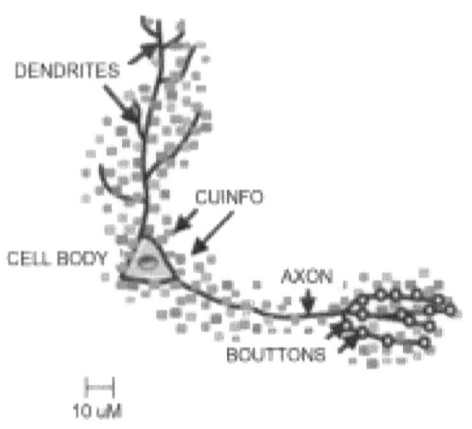

Fig. 9.7

- ◉ The figure shows the nECM surrounding a neuron. Neurons interact with the nECM with

dopants (metallic traces and neurotransmitters) that represent 'cognitive information units' (cuinfo).
  - [nECM] interactive neuroscience journal

- ◉ The protein synthesis and DNA/RNA elongation rates are too slow to serve as effectors of neuronal memory, which must be faster than 100 ms, at least for short-term memory.

- ◉ Structural modifications of the synapse do not explain the formation of short-term memory. It is expected that the encoding/decoding process at the molecular scale should be faster than the neuronal activation rate (< 100 ms).
  - [nECM] interactive neuroscience journal

- ◉ The nECM in the adult brain represents approximately 20% of its total volume. In vitro, studies have shown that nECM is essential in the accelerated formation of neuronal networks and their response.
  - [scientific reports] nature magazine

ATP Batteries

◉ *"Rechargeable molecular batteries that energize all cells."*

10.1 Introduction

- ◉ Reflections on ATP batteries:
- ◉ A battery is a source of energy.
- ◉ ATP (adenosine triphosphate) is a molecule that behaves like a tiny rechargeable battery. Each of our cells contains about a billion ATP molecules. ATP is the most important source of our mechanical and chemical energy. The figure shows its molecular model.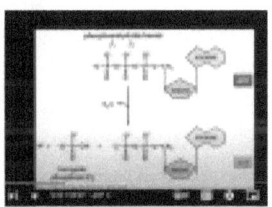
  - [ATP] [ATP molecular model] [molecular model] wikipedia

  - ◉ The following video by Chris Schubert (professor at Harvard and MIT) is an excellent presentation of the structure and importance of ATP as the source of life.
    - [ATP the source of life] youtube

- ◉ ATP is like a rechargeable battery; when it releases some of its energy, it is chemically converted into ADP. The figure shows its molecular model. When ADP is recharged, it is converted back to ATP.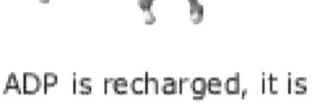
  - [ADP] [ADP molecular model] wikipedia

- ⊕ ATP batteries are recharged through the ingestion of food.
- ⊕ The release of energy from ATP batteries is used to construct the main bio-structures that allow life to exist, such as membranes, vesicles, DNA, RNA, and proteins. It is used to supply energy to molecular robots that are responsible for moving cargo within cells; It is used to generate the electricity needed by the neurons of our nervous system; It is used to energize our muscles, which are the essence of our motor functions that give our body all its movements; and many more things.

- ⓘ⊕ A biobot is a biological robot that performs a specialized and necessary job in some part of our body.
- ⊕ ATP batteries are underpinned by an energy generator, the ATP-Synthase biobot, which is used to generate ATP.
  - [ATP-synthase] [ATP] [molecular motor] wikipedia

    - ⊕ The figure video shows the ATP-Synthase biobot in action:
      - [Electron Transport Chain] youtube
    - ⊕ The ATP-Synthase biobots are densely packed in the inner mitochondrial membrane, making its entire surface a giant cellular power plant.

- ⊕ In 1948, ATP was first synthesized by Scottish biochemist Alexander Todd. In 1957, he received the Nobel Prize in part for his research on the structure and synthesis of ATP.
  - [alexander todd] wikipedia

    - ⊕ *The Nobel Prize in Chemistry • 1957, was awarded to Lord (Alexander R.) Todd "for his work on nucleotides and nucleotide coenzymes."*
      - [1957 Nobel Prize in Chemistry] nobelprize.org

Rings of the Mind

- ⊕ In 1957, Jens Christian Skou discovered the ATPase biobot used to transport ions. In 1997, he received the Nobel Prize in part for this work.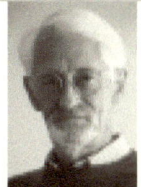
  - [jens christian skou] wikipedia

  - ⊕ *The Nobel Prize in Chemistry - 1997 was divided; part was awarded to Jens C. Skou for the first "discovery of an ion-transporting enzyme, $Na+$, $K+$ -ATPase.*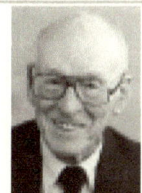
    - [1997 Nobel Prize in Chemistry] nobelprize.org

- ⊕ In 1974, Paul Boyer presented a theory that explained how ATP synthase works. In 1997, he received the Nobel Prize in part for this work.
  - [paul boyer] wikipedia

  - ⊕ *The Nobel Prize in Chemistry - 1997 was divided; part was awarded to Paul D. Boyer for his "elucidation of the enzymatic mechanism underlying the synthesis of ATP."*
    - [1997 Nobel Prize in Chemistry] nobelprize.org

- ⊕ In 1978, British biochemist Peter Mitchel received the Nobel Prize for his theory of the mechanism that explains ATP formation by moving hydrogen ions across a membrane during cellular respiration or photosynthesis.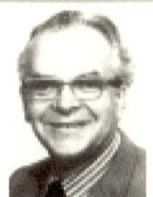
  - [peter mitchel] [chemiosmosis] wikipedia

  - ⊕ *The 1978 Nobel Prize in Chemistry was awarded to Peter D. Mitchell "for his contribution to the understanding of biological energy transfer through the formulation of chemiosmotic theory."*
    - [978 Nobel Prize in Chemistry] nobelprize.org

- ⊕ In 1994, John Walker used X-ray crystallography to determine the structure of ATP synthase. In 1997, he received the Nobel Prize in part for this work.

eduardo padilla-diaz

ZPUs

"Molecular processors that execute bio-software resulting in chemical transformations."

11.1 Introduction

- Reflections on ZPUs (enZimatic Processing Units):
- In the world of computers, there is a special machine called the CPU (Central Processing Unit), controlled by a master oscillator. The CPU executes sequences of software instructions that make countless useful informatic transformations.
  - [CPU] [software] wikipedia

  - When starting a computer, a voltage source supplies it with energy. A 'master oscillator' starts up and keeps the CPU active, which is responsible for executing the instruction sequences of its software at the rate of that master oscillator. At startup, its instruction pointer (IP) points to a fixed location, where the first instructions of the software are, which are responsible for initializing its OS operating system, and then begin to execute the functional instructions, which give it utility and purpose to the computer.
    - [IP] [OS] [hardware] wikipedia
  - This 'master oscillator' that starts and maintains the execution of instructions in a computer is like its soul.
- Similarly, in molecular biology, special machines called ZPUs (enZimatic Processing Units) are controlled by master oscillators. ZPUs execute sequences of

software instructions, which are used to make countless useful chemical and mechano-chemical transformations.
- [biología molecular] wikipedia

- ◉ When starting a molecular robot, an ATP source supplies it with energy. A 'master oscillator' starts up and keeps the ZPU active, which is responsible for executing the instruction sequences of its software at the rate of that master oscillator. At startup, its instruction pointer (IP) points to a fixed location, where the first instructions of the software are, which are responsible for initializing its OS operating system, and then begin to execute the functional instructions, which give it utility and purpose to the molecular robot.

- ◉ This 'master oscillator' that starts and maintains the execution of instructions in a molecular robot is like its soul.

Clocks

⚛ "All cells have a clock synchronized by a central clock in the brain."

12.1 Introduction

- ⚛ Reflections on biological clocks:
- ⚛ Who would have imagined that all the cells in the body have a clock and that a central clock in the brain synchronizes all these cellular clocks? This central clock, in turn, is synchronized with the circadian rhythm by special cells found in the eye.

  Here, we will explore circadian rhythm, central clock, cellular clocks, and cardiac clock:

1. ⚛ The circadian rhythm is any process in an organism that falls into a 24-hour rhythm or cycle.
   - [circadian rhythm] wikipedia

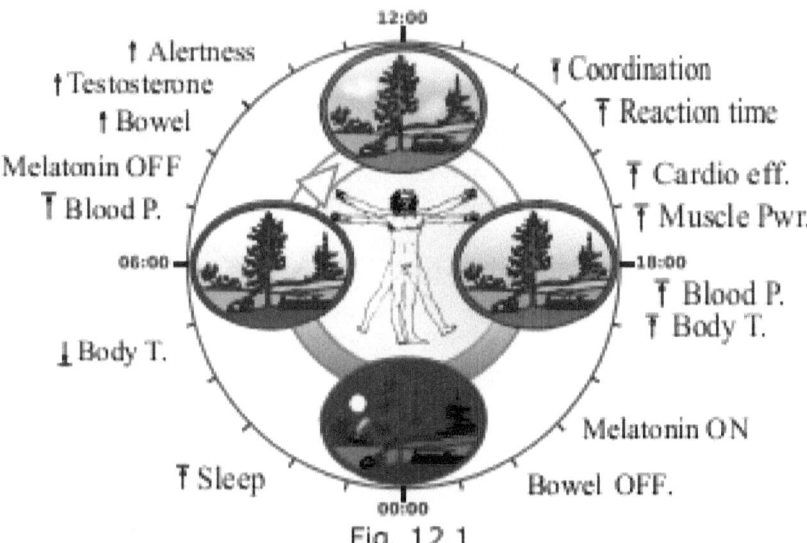

Fig. 12.1

- ⊕ The previuos figure shows how the circadian rhythm regulates the sleep-wake cycle and repeats itself with each rotation of the Earth approximately every 24 hours.
    - [Biological clock human] wikimedia
- ⊕ *The 2017 Nobel Prize in Physiology or Medicine was awarded to Jeffrey C. Hall, Michael Rosbash, and Michael W. Young, for their discoveries of the molecular mechanisms that control the circadian rhythm.*
    - [2017 Nobel Prize in Physiology or Medicine] nobelprize.org

---

- ⊕ The central clock is located in a small brain region called the SCN in the hypothalamus. It comprises about 20,000 neurons, receives direct information from the eyes, and controls and synchronizes the circadian rhythm of the entire body.
    - [SCN] [hypothalamus] wikipedia [central clock] Cambridge University Press

- ⊕ In the back of the eye, special photoreceptor cells called ipRGCs that, as soon as they detect light, message it to the SCN.
    - [ipRGC] wikipedia

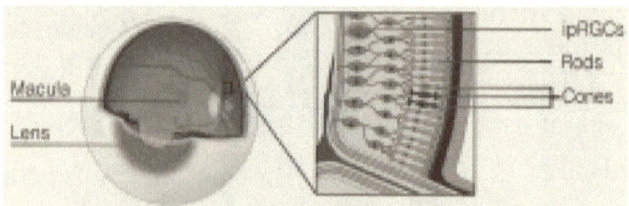

Fig. 12.2

- ⊕ The figure shows the placement of the ipRGC photoreceptors in the eye.
    - [Overview of the retina photoreceptors] wikimedia
- ⊕ As soon as the SCN receives the message that the light has been detected, it sends a message to all the

cells so that they can synchronize their rhythms with the SCN's circadian rhythm.

- ⚛ Cellular clocks: In the body, each cell has its own clock based on the levels of a protein called PER. PER helps establish the circadian rhythm within the cell. PER is synthesized from a gene known as Period. The SCN sets the circadian rhythm of each cellular clock to the correct time each day.
  - [PER] wikipedia

- ⚛ The heart clock determines the heart rate. Inside the heart, a small module of pacemaker cells generates electrical impulses that define the heart rate and travel through the heart's electrical conduction system, causing its contraction.
  - [heart rate] [pacemaker cells] wikipedia
  - The figure shows how the final shape of an ECG is made out of the shapes from different sources in the heart.
    - [Shapes of the cardiac action potential in the heart] wikimedia

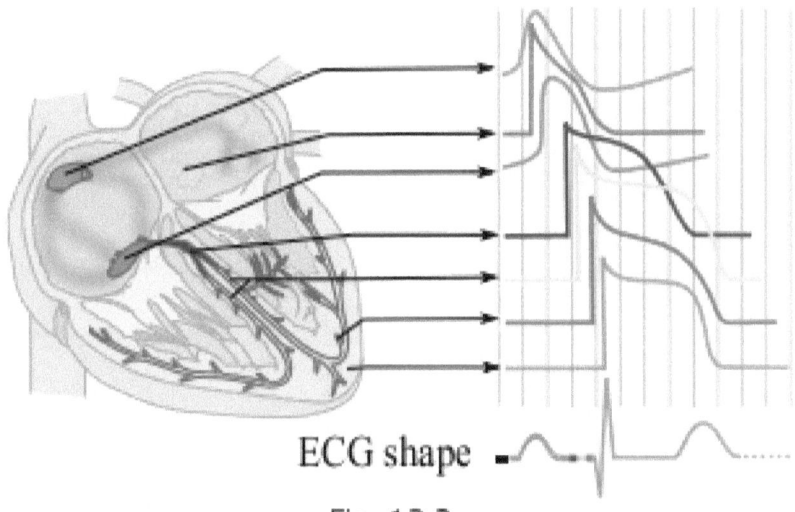

Fig. 12.3

eduardo padilla-diaz

Life

① *"Intelligent energy is transferred at the cellular level to create life at the human level."*

13.1 Introduction

- ◉ Reflections on life:
- ①◉ Life! that inexplicable form of intelligent energy that has been elusive to our understanding but expresses itself through our existence.
  1. ①◉ Since our pre-embryonic phase, life is responsible for creating our body and mind.
  2. ①◉ When we are born, life takes care of us internally. But our bodies are still very fragile, and our mental and motor skills are insufficient to protect us in the new outside world; then, something magical happens. The first time we connect sensorially with our parents, they change their goals and dedicate a large part of their lives to feeding, educating, and protecting us during the childhood stage of our external existence.
  3. ◉ That is why, during the first months of our external existence, life ensures that we cry so that we can be cared for, protected, and fed; that we begin to learn and respond to affection with a tender look or a sweet smile; and that we sleep up to 22 hours a day, in periods of two to five hours, so that while we rest, we strengthen and grow at an accelerated rate.
  4. ◉ As the days go by, life ensures that we grow, develop, and continue learning to acquire skills in all our motor movements to feed ourselves, move around,

and communicate to become autonomous in the home environment. At the same time, we show the progress of our physical and mental development.

5. ◉ In the first years of our childhood, life encourages us to play with striking objects that, thanks to our imagination, we virtually convert into infantile people, animals, and things. We begin to learn to communicate with signs and our first words. We begin to express with primitive pictures how we see our parents and surroundings.

6. ◉ Life ensures that we continue to improve and learn to become autonomous in the habitat where we operate. We can move safely between points of interest, find food and shelter, communicate with other human beings, entertain ourselves, and exchange information that benefits us.

7. ◉ When we reach the age of 10 to 12, puberty begins, and our bodies change to enable us to have children. Life also changes our minds and awakens in us the maximum attraction and desire to find an appropriate partner to reproduce by the selection imprinted by nature, in our genes, and imprinted on our minds by our experiences.

8. ◉ When we find a partner, life ensures that we fall in love to make it easier for us to mate, but it also gives us the chance to refrain from having children if we are not yet prepared for such responsibility.

9. ◉ Eventually, the day comes when we have improved ourselves enough, when love and passion meet, and we get to have children, thus achieving the transfer of life and the improvement of the species, which are among the primary purposes of life.

10. ⊕ And so, through the years, life ensures that we continue to improve and learn, to raise and educate our children well so that they can become autonomous, and thus guarantee the continuity of their existence and the preservation of the species, which is another of the primary purposes of life.

- ⊕ Next, we will explore life in space-time, life phases, and cellular life.

13.2 Life in space-time

- !⊕ Life in the domain of space-time has been elucidated thanks to the accumulation of human knowledge, the discovery of fossils of certain types of bacteria (cyanobacteria) more than 3.5 billion years old, and advances in TEM (2D) and SEM (3D) electron microscopy, which has allowed the study of said fossils and have allowed the study of matter on the scale of 0.2 nanometers; to the appearance of femtochemistry (4D) that has allowed us to study the behavior of atoms in chemical reactions, on the scale of femtoseconds; and the appearance of attophysics and atto-spectroscopy, which have allowed us to study the behavior of electrons at the atomic level, on the scale of attoseconds; all this, allowing us, in turn, to investigate in detail the fundamental processes of life.
  - [cyanobacteria] [TEM] [SEM] [femtochemistry] [femtosecond] [attophysics] [atto-spectroscopy] [attosecond] wikipedia [ultrafast science] scitechdaily

  1. ⊕ With the advent of TEM and SEM electron microscopes, the physical barrier of optical microscopes in the 200nm space reached 0.5nm and 0.2nm, respectively.

The figure/video created by PaperPen Biology shows how SEM generates 3D images. In addition, it explains the differences 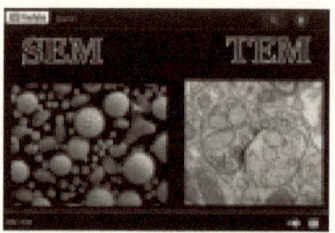 between the technologies, how these microscopes are made, their advantages, and their differences.
- [TEM vs SEM] youtube : PaperPen Biology

2. ⊕ In 1931, TEM was demonstrated by Max Knoll and Ernst Ruska, and this group developed the first TEM with greater than light resolution in 1933 and the first commercial TEM in 1939. In 1986, Ruska received the Nobel Prize in Physics for developing transmission electron microscopy.

   - ⊕ *The 1986 Nobel Prize in Physics was split: half was awarded to Ernst Ruska "for his fundamental work in electron optics and the design of the first electron microscope" and the other half jointly to Gerd Binnig and Heinrich Rohrer "for their design of the tunneling microscope."*
   - [1986 Nobel Prize in Physics] nobelprize.org

3. ⊕ Femtochemistry is the area of physical chemistry that studies chemical reactions in real-time on femtosecond scales. In 1988, Ahmed Hassan Zewail published an article using this 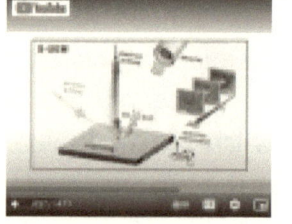 term for the first time in the journal Science. Later, in 1999, Zewail received the Nobel Prize in Chemistry for his pioneering work in this field. He demonstrated that it is possible to see how atoms move in a molecule during a chemical reaction.
   - [femtochemistry] youtube : NeoCairo

   - ⊕ *The 1999 Nobel Prize in Chemistry was awarded to Ahmed H. Zewail "for his studies of the transition*

states of chemical reactions using femtosecond spectroscopy."
- [1999 Nobel Prize in Chemistry] nobelprize.org

4. ⚛ Atto-spectroscopy won the 2023 Nobel Prize in Physics; it uses light pulses in the attosecond range to study and control the movement of electrons in atoms and 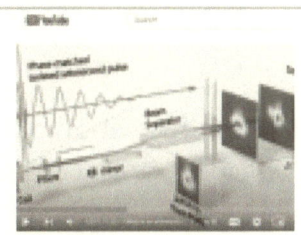 molecules, which are responsible for most of the matter's physical and chemical properties. Atto-spectroscopy has also helped reveal some of the secrets of the quantum world and the wonders of the cosmos. Let's consider that the fastest chemical reaction takes 1 femtosecond; 1 attosecond is 1000 times faster than a femtosecond; 1 attosecond is to a second, what a second is to 31 billion years (more than twice the age of the universe).
- [atto-spectroscopy] youtube

   - ⚛ *The 2023 Nobel Prize in Physics was awarded to Pierre Agostini, Ferenc Krausz, and Anne L'Huillier "for experimental methods generating attosecond pulses of light for the study of the dynamics of electrons in matter."*
   - [2023 Nobel Prize in Physics] nobelprize.org

13.3 Vital Phases

- 🌓 The formation of human beings has resulted from an evolution of vital matter through multiple phases, which are directly related to the rings of the mind and can be summarized in the following vital phases: vital matter, vital beings, living beings, and human beings.

- 🌓 The following table shows the relationship that exists between the rings of the mind and the vital phases:

mind rings	they form	has vital matter	has vital beings	has living beings	has humans	autonomous
atomic	atoms	no	no	no	no	no
molecular	biomolecules	Yes	no	no	no	no
molecular robots	RNA, ribozymes, viroids	Yes	Yes	no	no	no
protocellular RNA	RNA protocells	Yes	Yes	Yes	no	Yes
protocellular DNA	DNA protocells	Yes	Yes	Yes	no	Yes
prokaryotic cell	bacteria, archaea, viruses	Yes	Yes	Yes	no	Yes
organular	organelles	Yes	Yes	Yes	no	no
eukaryotic cell	eukaryotic cells	Yes	Yes	Yes	no	no
organic	organs and tissues	Yes	Yes	Yes	no	no
organic systems	organic systems	Yes	Yes	Yes	no	no
virtual	virtual organs	Yes	Yes	Yes	no	no
human	humans	Yes	Yes	Yes	Yes	Yes
external	groups, social networks	no	no	no	Yes	no

- 🛈 Below, the vital phases are described in more detail: vital matter, vital beings, living beings, and human beings.

  1. 🛈 Vital matter phase:
     - 🛈 Vital matter emerges in the ring of the molecular mind. It was initially made up only of RNA macromolecules, and from this, two different forms of macromolecules were generated: DNA and proteins.
       - [RNA] [DNA] [proteins] wikipedia
     - 🛈 These three macromolecules, RNA, DNA, and proteins, constitute the three forms of vital matter essential for all known life forms.
       - [RNA World] wikipedia

  2. 🛈 Vital beings phase:
     a. 🛈 Wells or special propitious environments in nature meet the physical, chemical, conducive, and other requirements for generating primitive vital beings from vital matter.
     b. 🛈 In a propitious environment, the first vital beings emerge from sequences of vital RNA matter—in an inexplicable way.
     c. 🛈 The propitious environment in which these vital beings are hosted allows them to develop, improve, and self-replicate, and these conditions are nothing less than the essence of evolution.
        - [evolution] wikipedia
          - 🛈 Vital beings are not autonomous because, to survive, they need a host.
          - 🛈 From now on, we will call these vital beings molecular robots.

d. 🛈⊕ These first molecular robots will evolve and form the first ribozymes and the first viroids.
   - [ribozymes] wikipedia [ribozymes] chemistry world

e. 🛈⊕ These molecular robots will evolve and join together with others to benefit from each other's services. More useful and robust infrastructures emerge from this mutual collaboration, with more powerful defense and feeding mechanisms allowing them to develop, improve, and self-replicate, giving rise to the first macro-molecular robots.

f. 🛈⊕ These macro-molecular robots will evolve and learn to encapsulate themselves in membranes with aqueous content, providing them with the necessary propitious environment and protection to become autonomous.

3. 🛈⊕ Living beings phase:

a. 🛈⊕ The evolution of these autonomous molecular macro robots will give rise to the first monocellular living beings: RNA protocells.
   - [Proto cells: at the interface of life and the nonliving] nlm.nih.gov

      - ⊕ The figure shows what could have been an RNA protocell, consisting mainly of a bilipid membrane, a string of RNA nucleotides containing the genome, ribozymes, and other components necessary for converting food to fuel, and in its self-replication

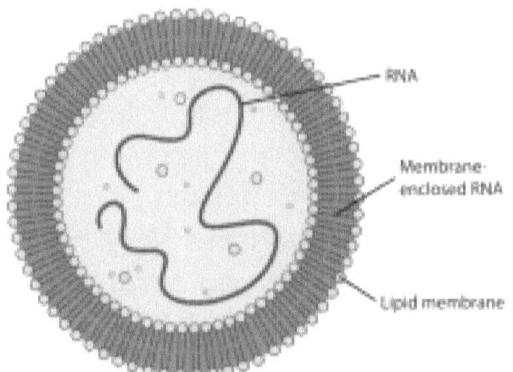

Fig. 13.1

b. 🌀 RNA protocells will evolve, thanks to their molecular robots and the evolution of the functionality of their groups. Some will learn to store the genome in DNA. Others will create the mechanism for extracting DNA into RNA to not affect the existing translation functionality. Others are going to begin to use a new, much more sophisticated form of vital matter based on chains of amino acids, and this will lead to the creation of much more rigid and complex infrastructures used to assemble tracks used for the transport of materials and to be able to control the shape and rigidity of their protective membranes; and, these RNA protocells will give rise to the appearance of DNA protocells.
- [proteins] wikipedia

c. 🌀 DNA protocells, whose genome is now entirely of double-stranded DNA chains, will provide a more stable storage medium and allow longer sequences. They will learn to make molecular robots based on amino acids, which are much more powerful and efficient. They will be able to create the infrastructure with the help of tracks and molecular robots to change the external shape of their protective cover to move in the environment where they are immersed.

They will evolve and create flagella motors to propel them more efficiently. They will make much more sophisticated protective membranes, with defense mechanisms capable of detecting the type of attacker. They will learn to remember how to defend themselves against these. They will be able to orient themselves and navigate the environment where they operate to search for objects of interest. They will evolve and give rise to the appearance of bacteria and archaea, known as prokaryotic cells.

d. 🔹🔸 Symbiogenesis (endosymbiotic theory, or serial endosymbiotic theory) is the leading evolutionary theory of the origin of eukaryotic cells from prokaryotic organisms. It has been deduced through genetic analysis that mitochondria could have been derived from a common ancestor that originated from integrating a certain type of endosymbiotic bacteria with an archaea-type host cell.

- [Symbiogenesis] wikipedia

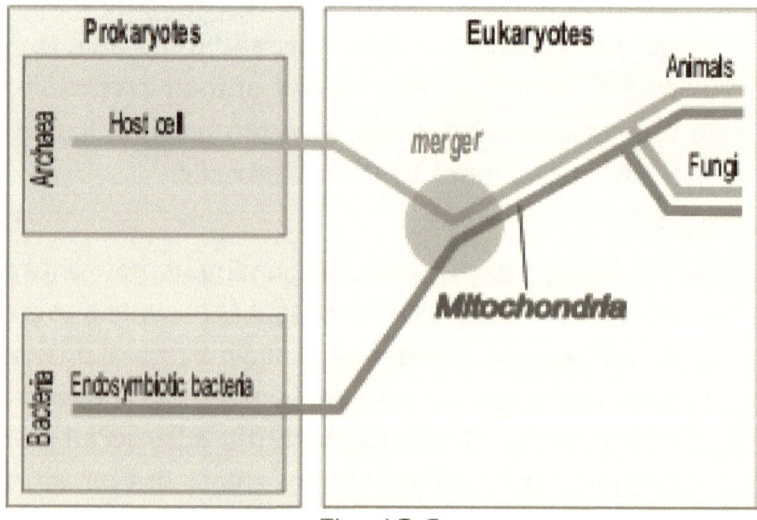

Fig. 13.2

e. ①◆ The archaeal cells, with their ribosomes, which are more sophisticated than those of their counterparts in bacteria, plus the endosymbiotic addition of mitochondria, will evolve and begin to outline much more sophisticated cells that will come to have many specialized organelles, such as the Golgi apparatus. These will give rise to the first multi-organelle cells known as eukaryotic cells.
    - [archaea : morphology] ucmp.berkeley.edu

f. ①◆ Then, these multi-organular mono-cellular living beings will evolve and give rise to multi-organic multi-cellular living beings, starting with fish, monotremes, marsupials, eutherians, and, finally, ending with human beings.

4. ①◆ Human beings phase:

    a. ①◆ In this phase, humans are formed.

13.4 Cellular Life

- ①◆ In the human body, cellular life is not created; it is transferred through the union of two living unicellular bodies: an egg and a sperm; both are genetically semicomplete, but when joined, they intertwine their genetic sequences, resulting in the mutation of the egg into a cell body with a complete genetic code. Then, through the mechanism of cellular reproduction, the cellular mind, with the help of its genetic knowledge, uses it to create all the organs of the body until forming the complete organic system of a human being capable of cradling the human mind, thus creating, in the end, human life.

- ⊕ The cell is the smallest organism that can be considered alive. There are unicellular organisms such as bacteria. There are also pluricellular organisms, such as the human body, which contains 37 trillion cells. In the human body, there are only two types of cells: somatic and reproductive.

1. ⊕ Somatic cells: They encompass almost all the cells in the body, and their primary function is to form tissues and, in some cases, replace dead cells.
    a. ⊕ The human body contains more than 200 different types of somatic cells, for example, neurons, epithelial cells, and leukocytes, which are found in the nervous system, skin, and blood, respectively.
    b. ⊕ Although somatic cells are very diverse in their form and function, they are all identical genetically because they do not express all their genes, only those of the cell group to which they belong. This process is called cellular differentiation, which occurs from the embryonic stage. Thus, certain genes are active in some cells and inactive in others. Because somatic cells do not participate in sexual reproduction, mutations can affect the individual but are not transmitted to their offspring
    c. ⊕ Somatic cells are diploid, meaning they have two sets of homologous chromosomes in their nucleus: one inherited from the father and the other from the mother.
        - [chromosomes] wikipedia
    d. ⊕ Somatic cells reproduce by mitosis, where two diploid cells are produced from one diploid cell, genetically equal to the cell of origin. The function of mitosis is to replace dead cells and form tissues.
        - [mitosis] wikipedia

e. ⊕ *The 2001 Nobel Prize in Physiology or Medicine was awarded jointly to Leland H. Hartwell, Tim Hunt, and Sir Paul M. Nurse "for their discoveries of key cell cycle regulators."*

- The cell cycle is the process that involves the growth of a cell, DNA synthesis, and mitosis to produce two daughter cells.

- [2001 Nobel Prize in Physiology or Medicine] nobelprize.org

2. ⊕ Reproductive cells have the purpose of creating new human beings through fertilization; they are made up of eggs and spermatozoids.

   a. ⊕ Eggs: They only exist in women and are found in their ovaries; the woman is born with all the eggs, she will produce ~ 6 million, and when she reaches puberty, she only has ~ 300,000 left.

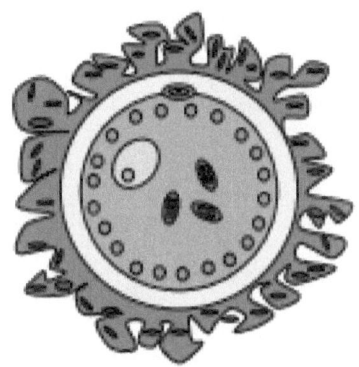

Fig. 13.3

The previous figure shows an illustration of the woman's egg. An egg can be fertilized by sperm and has a single set of chromosomes inherited from the mother in its nucleus.

- [egg cells] wikipedia [Ovum Diagram] wikimedia

b. ⊕ Spermatozoids only exist in men. They begin to be generated from 10 to 12 years of age; millions are produced daily in the testicles. They take approximately three months to mature; a fertile man can ejaculate between 15 and 250 million spermatozoids. The function of spermatozoids is to fertilize the female egg.
- [spermatozoids] wikipedia

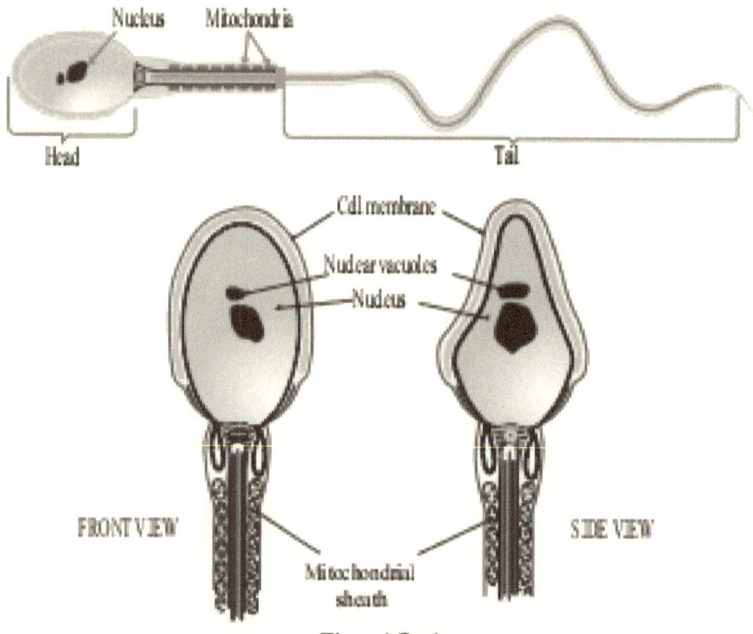

Fig. 13.4

- The figure shows in detail the structure of a spermatozoid cell.
  - [Complete diagram of a human spermatozoa] wikimedia

c. ⊕ Fertilization consists of a spermatozoid's fusion with an egg's nucleus, resulting in a zygote that will later give rise to the embryo and fetus. All cells resulting from the proliferation of the zygote

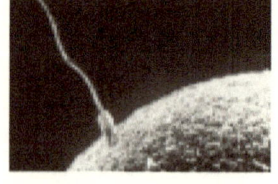

have the same genetic information but undergo cellular differentiation.
- [fertilization] wikipedia [Sperm-egg] wikimedia

- ◆ Cell differentiation occurs when a stem cell becomes a more specialized cell type. It occurs numerous times during the development of a multicellular organism as it changes from a simple zygote to a complex system of tissues and cell types. With a few exceptions, cell differentiation almost never involves a change in the DNA itself. Thus, different cells can have very different physical characteristics despite having the same genome.
  - [cell differentiation] [stem cell] wikipedia [Final stem cell differentiation] wikimedia

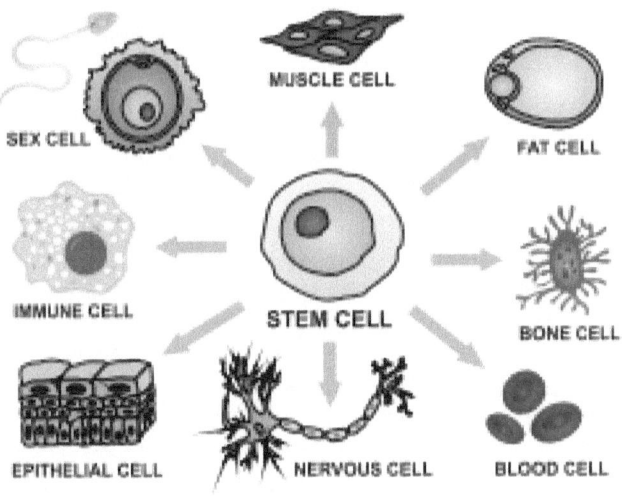

Fig. 13.5

eduardo padilla-diaz

Inconscience

* *"Aggregate functionality of all the minds below the virtual mind."*

14.1 Introduction

- ⬥ Reflections on the *Inconscience*:
- ⬥ *Inconscience* is a functional domain of the body that is out of reach of the consciousness of the virtual ring. In the virtual ring and above, we are unaware of what is happening in that domain.
- ⬥ *Inconscience* is not a centralized entity; we will not find it in a specific place in the body. On the contrary, *Inconscience* is distributed throughout the entire body.
- ⬥ *Inconscience* results from the aggregate functioning of those hundreds of millions of minds, found below the ring of the virtual mind, all working concurrently, guaranteeing that what is under the control of their minds works perfectly according to their purposes.
- ⬥ Let us consider that, in the body: behind every molecular robot, there is a molecular mind; behind every organelle, there is an organelle mind; behind every cell, there is a cellular mind; behind every organ, there is an organic mind; and so forth. The aggregate functionality of all those minds is what makes the *Inconscience*.
- ⬥ Certain gradual processes in our body are also part of the *Inconscience*. They are embedded in our genetics and manifest late in our development. It is important to know that they exist, and here we will only discuss puberty, which is briefly described below, and

externalization, which is described in the lingua mentis chapter.

- ◦ 🕮 Puberty: It is a gradual process that takes us out of childhood and prepares us for reproduction, which is, after nutrition, one of the vital functions that guarantee the preservation of our species. Puberty takes many years to begin and takes some time to complete. It is not convenient for our species that we are ready to reproduce early because, in the first years of our life, we need more knowledge, maturity, or strength to face having children. That is why the process of puberty appears when we have already acquired sufficient knowledge, sufficient maturity, and sufficient strength to be able to face the changes that we will be subject to in this gradual process, during which we will be subject to extreme and necessary changes, to prepare for procreation properly; and so that at the end of this process, we are in optimal conditions, both physically and mentally, to generate strong and healthy children; and as a result, guarantee their well-being and appropriate development, and the continuity of our species.
    - [puberty] wikipedia

Objects of Interest

"The most transcendental concept in capturing useful sensory information."

15.1 Introduction

- Reflections on the objects of interest:
- The objects of interest, in the context of the mind, are the most transcendental and important concept in understanding the thinking system; without them, we couldn't explain it.
    - The objects of interest are in the human mind, the representation of instances of people, animals, plants, and things.
    - The objects of interest are in the animal mind, the representation of instances of members of the same species, other animals, plants, and things.
    - From the sensory point of view, objects of interest are multimodal since different sensory centers can detect them.
        - Example: When a dog barks, our acoustic center detects the sound of its barking, and concurrently, our visual center detects the image of the dog.
    - The objects of interest facilitate the extraction of the useful information they generate. That information is manifested through attributes of space, time, emotion, and affection, packaged in thinking messages sent to the thinking system for processing.

- 🕐◆ Space attributes such as position, orientation, size (if visual), volume (if acoustic), and more.
- 🕐◆ Time attributes such as motion, the direction of motion in space, and whether they are moving away or toward us.
- 🕐◆ Emotion attributes: such as their facial expression of happiness.
- 🕐◆ Affection attributes such as the affection evoked in a cub towards his mother.

• 🕐◆ A 'new' human mind has no acquired knowledge; therefore, it resorts to innate knowledge and abstraction so that our thinking can abstractly process the objects of interest from our prenatal phase. To clarify this, we need to consider the following terms: abstraction, concept, class, template, prototype, and schema:

1. 🕐◆ Abstraction: is the process of extracting the essence that uniquely characterizes and identifies something.
   - [abstraction (software)] [abstraction] wikipedia

2. 🕐◆ Concept: is the mental representation of an abstraction.
   - ◆◆ Example: the silhouette of a dog is a visual concept that characterizes it and differentiates it from the rest of the animals.
   - ◆◆ Example: a dog's bark is an auditory concept that characterizes it and differentiates it from the rest of the animals.
   - 🕐◆ Concepts are grouped according to the sensory center that perceives them, so there are concepts such as visual, auditory, olfactory, virtual, and so on.

3. Class: is the abstract, real, or virtual representation of an object of interest.
    - Examples of abstract classes: person, animal, plant, thing.
    - Examples of real classes: father, dog, tree, house.
    - Examples of virtual classes: superman, snoopy, kryptonite.
4. Template: is the genetic representation of a class.
    - Our genetic code has at least the templates of the following abstract classes: person, animal, plant, and thing.
5. Prototype: is the biological expression of a template.
    - Our sensory centers have at least prototype templates of the abstract classes: person, animal, plant, and thing.
        - Thanks to these prototypes, the sensory centers can extract these objects of interest from the sensory fields, allowing the mind to understand and process them abstractly. Sensory fields are described later in the 'Fields' chapter.
        - As knowledge about a specific object of interest is acquired, its prototype becomes more specific, allowing the mind to process it in a particular way and correlate it easily with its acquired knowledge.
6. Schema: In the knowledge context, it encompasses the rules that govern a set of associated classes. It facilitates knowledge storage, accumulation, extraction, exchange, and processing through cognitive transactions. Here, we are only going to briefly

introduce the following types of schemas: semantic and events:

- ◆ Semantic: allows us to understand the thinking messages generated by the objects of interest. Thinking messages are cognitive microtransactions that the sensory centers send to the thinking center for processing. Thinking messaging is explored in detail later.

- ◆ Events allow us to store in knowledge the most important things that happened in the present so that we can remember and understand them in the future. Events are macro cognitive transactions at the level of understanding, which allow us to understand the relationship that the objects of interest had with time, space, and each other. Events are described later.

Lingua Mentis

"An innate mechanism of a language is embedded in our brain."

16.1 Introducción

- Reflections on linguistics (part 1):
- Who would have thought that how we express ourselves linguistically had its roots in how our mind communicates with its linguistic components. After all, if it weren't for that, it would be very difficult to explain why most natural languages have a common mechanism and structure; this could be attributed to a first language, or several, which were the mothers of all languages, but it would be impossible to explain how all these first languages branched, became independent, and evolved with such perfection; so that all of them, throughout their long existences, had so many things in common in their mechanism and structure.
- What is possible to accept - and which would support the above - is that the mechanism and structure of a language of the *mind* - or *lingua mentis* - has always been embedded in our brain and that it is the mechanism that the *mind* uses internally for communication between all its linguistic components, as are all those related to the thinking system.
    - And that by another mechanism also embedded in our brain, which we will call externalization - which is explained later - which has the main purpose of externalizing the *lingua mentis*, so that a lingua prima or several are created, which are the basis of all natural

languages so that we use them to communicate with each other; and that as they branch out and evolve, they continue to preserve the bases and principles of the *lingua mentis*, which was intelligently designed by the wise hand of our Creator.

- [semiology] [latin] [Romance languages] [lingua franca] [lmother tongue] [pantomime] wikipedia

16.2 Coding and Cognitive Particles

1. I would also dare to say that the symbology of the lingua mentis could be based on information similar to that obtained by our visual sensors. It could be something like a sensory mass from which a cognitive particle is extracted, containing at least two components: a sensory expression and a linguistic expression.

    a. The sensory expression represents the acquired focal image, where the object of interest is under the focus; this sensory expression is used by the thinking system with the help of the imagination to reproduce, when needed, the image of the object of interest and the sensation, virtually in the future.

    b. The thinking system uses the linguistic expression to understand the image of the object of interest and the sensation.

2. Transporting a sensory expression through the body's networks would be almost impossible since it would entail unnecessary consumption of the networks' capacity and energy and considerably degrade the thinking system response time. That is why the sensory expression is stored in a single place in memory, whether temporary or

permanent. A referential token - which we will call *sensory expression - is transported through the networks, which is very compact and allows us to find the sensory expression in memory quickly.

3. Although the above used the visual modality as an example, all our sensors present modal symbology, which allows them to identify inherently—and more clearly—the attributes and associativity of the acquired information. Still, it can be asserted that the coding of visual sensory expressions is not similar to the coding of auditory sensory expressions or any of the other sensory expressions produced by each modality.

    - Each sensory expression is encoded in the native language of the sensory center where it occurred.

4. Therefore, the sensory expression of a visual cognitive particle can only be reproduced by the visual imagination in the projector of the visual center since the sensory expression is encoded in a native visual language. The same occurs with a sensory expression of an auditory cognitive particle; this can only be reproduced by the auditory imagination in the projector of the auditory center since the sensory expression is encoded in a native auditory language, and so, in general, we can say:

    - The reproduction of sensory expressions is modal since they can only be reproduced by the imagination of the sensory center that produced them.

5. Instead, the linguistic expressions are encoded in *lingua mentis* and, therefore, are understandable by the different components of the *mind* that use them; this is how the thinking system can understand all types of

linguistic expressions coming from all its sources since they are expressed in the language of the *mind*.

- 🔵 Linguistic expressions are multi-modal and, therefore, are understandable by the different components of the *mind* that use them.

16.3 Externalización

- 🔵 Externalization is a gradual process embedded in our genetics and manifests late in our development. This process has the primary purpose of externalizing the internal mechanism of the language of the *mind*: The *lingua mentis*, so that we use it to communicate externally with others. The first step of the process consists of detecting whether we - as we grow and develop - have not been exposed to the teaching of external linguistics - such as acoustic linguistics or written linguistics; the *mind* easily detects this due to the lack of symbols in a certain part of our sensory vocabularies, where all the intralinguistic information is stored, associated with the translation between the *lingua mentis* and the external natural language (or external natural languages), which we use to communicate with others. Suppose there is a lack of information in the translation memory of the *lingua mentis*. In that case, the externalization process gradually triggers a series of phases to externalize the mechanics and structure of the *lingua mentis*. At the end of these phases, the result is the creation of a lingua prima, or natural language, structured according to our genetic code, with which we can communicate with a natural language, which is capable of describing everything there is, everything that is, everything that has been done, everything we have done, everything that has been, everything we have been, everything we would like to do; in itself, so that we communicate linguistically everything related to matter, space, and time, emotions, and spirit, where we are immersed. In addition to these benefits, creating the lingua prima based on the *lingua mentis* allows the *mind* to perceive external linguistic information with a minimum of conversion since the components of our linguistic messages are by the mechanics and structure of the *lingua mentis*. On the other hand, if, in the first step of externalization, the *mind* detects the presence of symbols in intralinguistic memory, the process considers accomplished its mission of generating a lingua prima; by then, we have been subject for a long time to learning the lingua prima, acquired by our parents or mentors, in charge of guiding us in its learning.

eduardo padilla-diaz

Vocabularies

◐ *"Learning machines that transform sensations into cognitive particles."*

17.1 Introduction

- ◆ Reflections on linguistics (part 2):
- ◐◆ Vocabularies are learning machines that help the sensory centers recognize objects of interest present in the sensory fields.
  - ◐◆ Vocabularies are modal, so the visual center only has visual vocabularies; the acoustic center only has acoustic vocabularies; and the same thing happens with the other sensory centers.
  - ◐◆ For a given modality, vocabularies are composed of an innate vocabulary and an acquired vocabulary:
    - ◐◆ The innate vocabulary is genetic and necessary; without it, we could not operate or function as soon as we were born. So, we can say:
      - ◐◆ The innate visual vocabulary contains prototypes of images that allow us to recognize people, animals, plants, and things within the visual field.
      - ◐◆ The innate visual vocabulary also contains image prototypes that allow animals to recognize within a visual field: those of their species.
      - ◐◆ The innate acoustic vocabulary contains prototypes of sounds that allow us to recognize

within an acoustic field: people, animals, plants, and things.

- 🛈 And the same thing happens with the other innate vocabularies of the different sensory centers.

- 🛈 The acquired vocabulary allows us to recognize objects of interest that have previously interested us and have been added to this vocabulary; for example:

    - 🛈 Before birth, the acquired acoustic vocabulary allows us to recognize acoustically our mother.

    - 🛈 After birth, the acquired olfactory vocabulary also allows us to recognize our mother by her odor.

    - 🛈 After birth, the acquired visual vocabulary allows us to recognize visually our mother, father, and other family members.

    - 🛈 Sometime after birth, the acquired visual vocabulary allows us to recognize visually our habitat, other people, animals, plants, and other things we have seen.

Fields

"Sensory fields (visual, acoustic, etc.) that excite the sensors of our sensory centers."

18.1 Introduction

- Reflections on sensory fields:
- Here, we will begin to explore the following: sensory field, sensory centers, visual center, visual fields, vocabularies, and objects of interest.

1. A sensory field is a modal energy field (visual, acoustic, etc.) created by the sum of the energies generated by all the sources that excite the sensors of a sensory center.

2. Sensory centers process sensory fields modally: the visual center only processes visual fields, the acoustic center only processes acoustic fields, and so do all the other sensory centers.

    - Although there are multiple sensory modalities, such as visual, acoustic, tactile, smell, and others, here we will focus on the visual modality, which is the most important and complete and serves as an example for understanding the other modalities.
    - The sensory centers pour the information they capture directly into their reality projectors, and they extract from it useful information that is poured into channels, such as the MP channel (channel of thinking messages) and in others, described later in the chapter: channels.

3. ◈ The visual center is a sensory center of the mind, where everything related to visual informatics is exclusively processed. This center is explored in detail later in several chapters, but we are only interested in considering the visual field.
    - ◈ A visual field represents all the light energy that excites our eyes at a given moment.
    - ◈ The visual field comprises several fields, but we will limit the exploration to the field of interest and the focus field.
        - ◈ The visual field of interest covers a spherical area extending more than 180 degrees; each visual meridian contains all objects of interest detected by the visual center.
            - ◈ Example: When we are driving a car, the following objects of interest could be present in the visual field of interest: the road in the front lane, the vehicle in front of our car, the rearview mirror, the rearview mirror on the left, the rearview mirror on the right, the speedometer on the dashboard, the warning signs that appear on the road, and the road in the left lane.
            - ◈ The set of objects in the visual field of interest at a given moment is called a scene.
            - ◈ When an interesting change occurs in an object of interest that does not have the focus, the visual center informs the visual attention center, which informs the conscience, which may reconsider which object of interest should have the focus.
                - ◈ The conscience controls the visual field of focus within the visual field of interest, usually in the

center. It covers a much smaller spherical area within the visual field and has higher resolution. It contains the object of interest that the conscience asked the visual center to bring into focus.

- ◆ For example, if the conscience asks the visual center to focus on the vehicle in front of the car, the focus field of view would contain that object of interest.

- ◆ When there is an interesting change in the object of interest under focus, the visual center detects it, transforms it, and sends it as a thinking message to the *thinker* for processing. The Thinking Messages are covered in detail in the next book of this series: The Width of the Present.

4. ◆◆ Vocabularies are learning machines that help the sensory centers recognize objects of interest present in the sensory fields.

5. ◆◆ Objects of interest are present in the sensory fields that the sensory centers can recognize as part of their vocabularies.

eduardo padilla-diaz

MC-1

⊕ *"The Motor Center 1 controls all our movements, from molecules to muscles."*

19.1 Introduction

- ⊕ Reflections on the motor centers:
- ⊕ Motor center (MC): is in charge of all the control and movement of the body's moving parts. The motor center is explored in several parts: MC-1, P-1, MC-2, and P-2:
  - ⊕ MC-1: explores the motor center at the molecular, organelle, cellular, and muscular levels. This center is explored below.
  - ⊕ P-1 presents the *thinker* system's first model and the motor center's first version at a functional level.
  - ⊕ MC-2: explores the motor center at an operational level. This center is explored in the second book of this series titled 'The Width of the Present.'
  - ⊕ P-2: presents a more advanced model of the *thinker* system and a more advanced version of the motor center at a functional level. It is explored in the second book in this series, 'The Width of the Present.'
- ⊕ Here, we explore MC-1: the motor center at the molecular, organelle, cellular, and muscular levels.
- ⊕ The motor centers are in charge of all the control and movement of all the moving parts of the body that we use consciously, subconsciously, and unconsciously to:

- ◉ Operate the entire vocal apparatus to: speak, chew, bite, kiss, caress, sing, lick, drink, whistle, gargle, blow, suck, spit, sneeze, cough, hold, laugh, smile, cry, and else.
- ◉ Operate all the muscles of the face and eyes to frown; open and close the eyelids; move and focus the eyes; control light intensity, tears, and more.
- ◉ Skillfully operate something with our hands, arms, and other body parts to write, paint, carve, sculpt, eat with utensils, etc.
- ◉ Play musical instruments, such as the piano and all types of keyboards; the guitar and all stringed instruments; the saxophone and all wind instruments; the marimba, and so on.
- ◉ Play percussion instruments, such as maracas, castanets, tambourines, bongos, timbales, drums, and others—xylophones and all wind instruments, the marimba, etc.
- ◉ Walking, running, jumping, climbing, swimming, skating, rowing, sliding, crawling, playing sports, riding a horse, riding a bicycle, driving a car, etc.
- ◉ And many more movements.

- ◉ Each motor center is an extraordinarily sophisticated machine capable of executing all types of movement control precisely, cleanly, and silently.
  - ◉ Each motor center self-lubricates, self-maintains, self-regenerates, and rebuilds itself.
  - ◉ Each motor center performs its functions autonomously, requiring minimal conscious intervention.

- ◉ As we will see later, the *thinker* system only sends high-level messages to each motor center, and each one executes them autonomously, isolating the *thinker* system from all the immense complexity that motor functions require to execute.
- ◉ Each motor center is so complex and sophisticated that it would take much time and wisdom to describe it in detail. We will limit ourselves to exploring the minimum necessary to understand its importance in this adventure.
- ◉ The motor centers comprise the ocular motor center, the vocal motor center, the facial motor center, the neck motor center, the trunk motor center, the motor centers of the upper extremities, the motor centers of the lower extremities, and others located within these. We will treat them in a unified way, as the motor center, since they all share much of what we will explore below.
- ◉ The following sections cover the motor center at the molecular, cellular, and muscular levels.

19.2 Motor Center - Molecular Level

- ◉ Myosin robots are a superfamily of molecular robots known for their role in muscle contraction and many other motility processes. They use ATP energy and convert it into movement or mechanical work.
  - [myo] [myosin] [ATP] wikipedia
  - ◉ The micrographs show a myosin II clearly as it is. (courtesy of David Shotton).
    - [micrograph] wikipedia

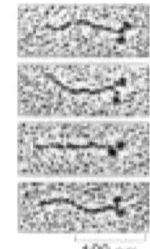

- ◉ The figure shows in detail the structure of a myosin II robot.
  - [myosin II] ncbi.nlm.nih.gov

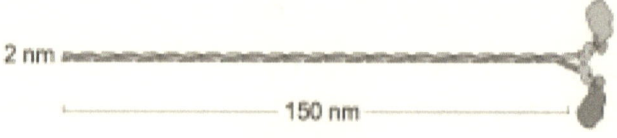

Fig. 19.1

- ◉ Consider that a myosin II robot moves in discrete steps, approximately 5 to 10 nanometers long, and generates a force of 1 to 5 pico newtons, the same force that gravity exerts on a single bacteria. This force will be used during muscle contraction.
  - [myosin: the actin motor protein] ncbi.nlm.nih.gov

- ◉ Myosin II robots assemble linearly in groups of ~250 to form robot filaments. These filaments operate on actin tracks, assisted by titin anchors, forming structures called sarcomeres.
  - [sarcomeres] wikipedia

- ◉ Sarcomeres are superstructures of robots specialized in muscle contraction. They are repeated along the muscle fibers, containing all the components to generate a distributed muscle contraction. The figure shows the basic composition of a sarcomere:
  - [Molecular Biology of the Cell. 4th edition] ncbi.nlm.nih.gov

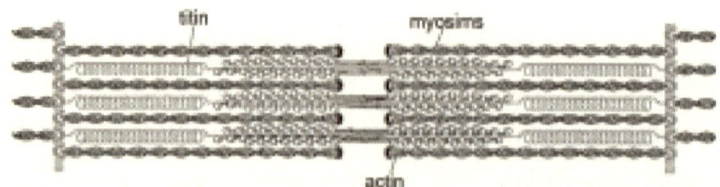

Fig. 19.2

- ○ ⊕ The myosin robots line up in groups to distribute their force. They grab the actin tracks to contract the muscle, and when they are released, the elastic titin anchor relocates them to their place of origin, relaxing the muscle.
    - [myosin] [actin] [titin] wikipedia
- ○ ⊕ The actin tracks guide the myosin robots to grip and walk to contract the muscle.
    - [actin] wikipedia
    - *Nomination for the Nobel Prize in Physiology or Medicine - 1957, to Albert von Szent-Gyorgyi Nagyrapolt for his discoveries in "muscle contraction and the role of myosin, actin, and ATP." Albert von Szent-Gyorgyi has been nominated 22 times.*
        - [1957 nomination for the Nobel Prize in Physiology or Medicine] nobelprize.org
    - ⊕ *The 1937 Nobel Prize in Physiology or Medicine was awarded to Albert von Szent-Gyorgyi Nagyrapolt "for his discoveries in relation to biological combustion processes, with special reference to vitamin C and the catalysis of fumaric acid."*
        - [1937 Nobel Prize in Physiology or Medicine] nobelprize.org

19.3 Motor Center - Cellular Level

- ⊕ Note: This exploration focuses exclusively on the muscle cells that make up skeletal muscles.
- ⊕ Skeletal muscle cells (muscle fibers), like most eukaryotic cells in the body, are composed of small organs called organelles, which we have previously explored. Here, we are only going to consider the particulars of these cells, such as their nuclei and the group of organelles made up of: the sarcolemma, the myofibrils, the sarcoplasmic reticulum, and the

transverse tubules, which form a sophisticated network of highly distributed channels, which facilitate the injection of calcium ions (Ca 2+) to all the sarcomeres that make up a large part of the cell body. Calcium ions are the particles that excite the sarcomeres to contract. One biceps brachii muscle cell can contain up to 80,000 sarcomeres.

1. ⦿ Myofibrils are rod-shaped organelles; they are composed of chains of sarcomeres.
   - [myofibril] wikipedia [Blausen 0801 Skeletal Muscle] wikimedia

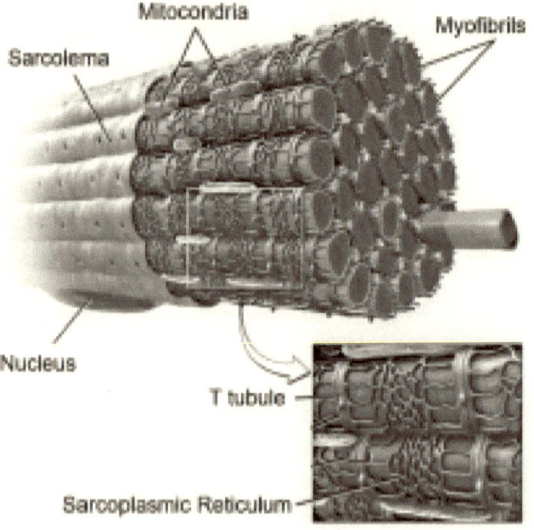

Fig. 19.3

- ⦿ The figure shows the interior of a skeletal muscle cell in detail. As can be seen, its content is made up of strips of myofibrils, and each of these - as we saw in the previous section - is full of sarcomeres.

2. ⦿ Sarcolemma is the membrane of a muscle cell; at each end, it fuses with a fiber of the tendon and the tendon fibers, joining together in bundles to form muscle tendons that adhere to the bones.
   - [sarcolemma] wikipedia

3. ⊕ The sarcoplasmic reticulum is a structure attached to the cell membrane that stores calcium ions (Ca 2+).
    - [Sarcoplasmic reticulum (2023, February 12)] wikipedia [1023 T-tubule] wikimedia

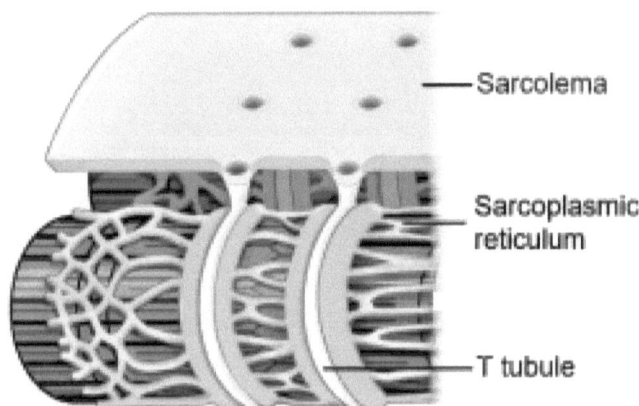

Fig. 19.4

4. ⊕ T-tubules are extensions of the cell membrane that allow rapid transmission of the action potential and also play an essential role in regulating cellular calcium concentration, allowing cells to contract more strongly by synchronizing the release of calcium throughout the cell.
    - [T-tubule] wikipedia

5. ⊕ The nuclei are distributed throughout the cell, and each has its domain responsible for supporting the volume of cytoplasm in that particular section. The nuclei are imprisoned against the sarcolemma, and each skeletal muscle cell can contain hundreds to thousands of nuclei to produce the large amounts of proteins and enzymes necessary for normal function. For example, a human bicep with a length of 10 cm can have up to 3000 nuclei.
    - [skeletal muscle] wikipedia

6. ⊕ Skeletal muscle cells are innervated by motor neuron synapses. The figure shows a muscle fiber innervated by a motor neuron. Soendenbroe, C., Andersen, J.L., & Mackey, A.L. (2021).
    - [American Journal of Physiology- Vol. 321, No. 2] journals.physiology.org

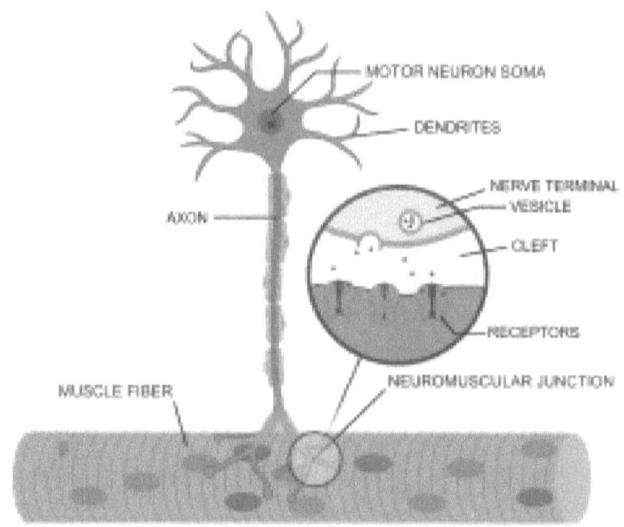

Fig. 19.5

19.4 Motor Center - Muscular Level

- ⊕ In general, muscles are made of muscle cells. They are structured to produce force and movement. They are primarily responsible for maintaining and changing posture and locomotion, as well as the movement of internal organs, such as the heart's contraction, and food through the digestive system. There are three types of muscles: skeletal, cardiac, and smooth. Here, we are only going to explore the skeletal muscles, the muscle spindles, and the Golgi tendon organ:
    - [muscles] wikipedia

- ◈ Skeletal muscles are made of muscle fascicles, which, in turn, are made of skeletal muscle cells (muscle fibers) wrapped by a type of connective tissue, as illustrated in the figure on the right.
    - [skeletal muscle] [muscle fascicle] wikipedia

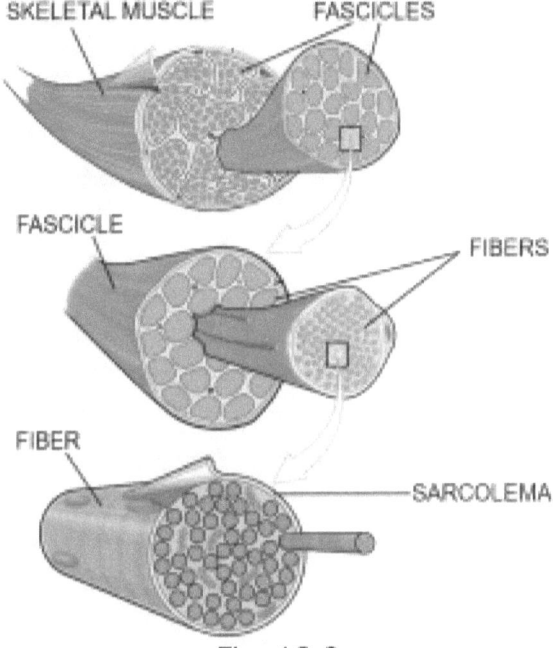

Fig. 19.6

- ◈ Muscle spindles are sensors within the body of a muscle that primarily detect changes in the length of the muscle. They transmit length information to the nervous system to give us the sensation of self-movement and body position, known as proprioception. They play an important role in regulating contraction to prevent muscle breakdown.
    - [muscle spindles] [central nervous system] [proprioception] wikipedia
        - ◈ The following figure shows how a muscular spindle has sensory and motor components. A description of how it works is found in its reference.

- [Muscle spindle model] wikimedia

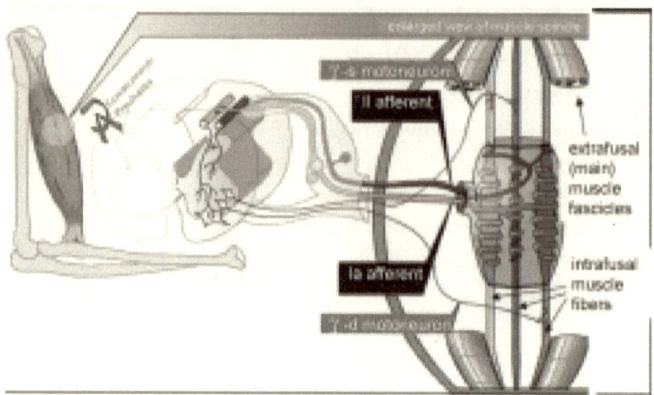

Fig. 19.7

- ✪ The Golgi tendon organ is a proprioceptive sensory receptor organ that helps regulate the tension that a muscle generates in the tendons so that they do not tear. It is found in the skeletal muscle tendons and provides the sensory component of the Golgi tendon reflex.
  - [golgi tendon organ] wikipedia

  - ✪ The following video by Kevin Tokoph clearly explains how the Golgi tendon organs and muscle spindles work together.

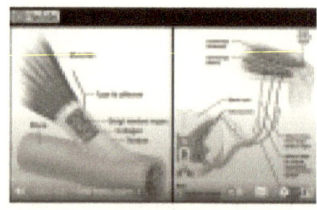

    - [anatomy and physiology of muscle spindles] youtube: Kevin Tokoph · catalyst university

- ✪ As an interesting fact, 1 cm of muscle cell can have from 120,000 to 450,000 sarcomeres.
  - [sarcomere] wikipedia

VC-1

⚜ *"The Visual Center 1 allows photons to show us visual reality."*

20.1 Introduction

- ⚜ Reflections on the visual center:
- ⚜ The visual center (VC) is a sensory center of the body, where everything related to visual information is exclusively processed. The visual center is explored in several parts: VC-1, P-1, VC-2, and P-2:
    - ⚜ VC-1: explores the visual center at the photon and sensory levels. This center is explored below.
    - ⚜ P-1 presents the *thinker* system's first model and the visual center's first version at a functional level.
    - ⚜ VC-2 explores the visual center at the operational level. The second book of this series, The Width of the Present, also explores this center.
    - ⚜ P-2 presents a more advanced model of the thinker system and a more advanced version of the visual center at a functional level. It is explored in the second book of this series, 'The Width of the Present.'

- ⚜ The visual center is the most important sensory center of the human being. From the moment we are born, we can recognize and differentiate abstractly people, animals, plants, and things through innate visual knowledge. As we grow, mature, and learn, the visual knowledge acquired increases, and with this, the capabilities of our visual center increase, such as:
    1. ⚜ It allows us to recognize our mother.

2. ◈ It allows us to recognize our loved ones.
3. ◈ It allows us to explore and learn the home environment.
4. ◈ It allows us to learn how to differentiate the colors and textures of matter.
5. ◈ It allows us to recognize, learn, and understand facial and body gestures.
6. ◈ It allows us to avoid collision with obstacles when learning to mobilize.
7. ◈ It allows us to explore, learn, and appreciate the habitat.
8. ◈ It allows us to recognize people, animals, plants, and things that can cause us harm.
9. ◈ It allows us to explore, learn, and appreciate clouds, mountains, vegetation, fruits, flowers, rivers, streams, lakes, the sea, meadows, and other members of nature.
10. ◈ It allows us to recognize insects, mammals, birds, fish, and other members of the animal kingdom.
11. ◈ It allows us to detect the gender, age, and beauty of the human beings and animals we see.
12. ◈ It allows us to recognize the sadness, wonder, joy, and more of the beings we interact with.
13. ◈ It allows us to communicate in writing, graphics, and signs with other humans.
14. ◈ It allows us to store information in written form or graphically in documents, portraits, videos, films, statues, monuments, and other persistent media.
15. ◈ It allows us to read books, documents, messages, and signs.

16. ⊕ It allows us to explore and learn the paths that lead us to points of interest.
17. ⊕ It has allowed us to create garments to shelter and dress ourselves.
18. ⊕ It has allowed us to create glasses, binoculars, microscopes, telescopes, screens, televisions, light bulbs, and many more augmented reality instruments.
19. ⊕ It has allowed us to create tools and utensils, such as knives, forks, plates, glasses, and more.
20. ⊕ It has allowed us to create transparent mediums, such as glass, to isolate ourselves from noise, temperature, humidity, pressure, wind, water, dangerous gases, vacuum, and other elements foreign to our favorable environment.
21. ⊕ It allows us to appreciate and learn art, architecture, fashion, ballet, decoration, and other manifestations of visual expression.
22. ⊕ It allows us to explore, appreciate, and learn about matter, the universe, the virtual, the past, the present, the future, the artificial, and everything we can capture with our visual center.

- ⊕ The visual center is a powerful machine that allows us to see and interact with the visual reality where we are.
  - ⊕ The conscience normally controls the visual center. But, as we will see later, some reflexes automatically control it in emergencies, and in semi-automatic situations, it is controlled by the subconscience.
  - ⊕ The visual center is made up mainly of two stereo visual detectors and a visual motor center.
    - ⊕ The two stereo-visual detectors are the retinas found on the inner back of each eye.

- ⊕ Each retina has approximately 100 million photoreceptor cells responsible for transmitting information simultaneously to the visual center for processing.
  - ⊕ The information captured by the eyes comprises two concentric parts: the focal visual field and the peripheral visual field.
  - ⊕ The visual motor center positions the head and each eye to a point of interest. It controls the focus and opening of each iris according to the amount of light to give us an image with the maximum possible clarity and sharpness in each eye.
- ⊕ Here, we explore the visual center VC-1 at the photon and sensory levels.

20.2 Visual center at the photon level

- ⊕ An elementary particle called the photon, the basic light unit, is the smallest discrete amount of electromagnetic radiation. Photons have no mass and move at the speed of light in a vacuum.
  - [fotón] wikipedia
- ⊕ In 1900, Max Planck suggested that energy carried by electromagnetic waves could only be released in discrete packets of energy, which he called 'quanta.'
  - [max planck] [cuantos] wikipedia

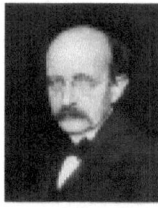

  - ⊕ *The 1918 Nobel Prize in Physics was awarded to Max Karl Ernst Ludwig Planck "in recognition of the*

services he rendered to the advancement of Physics through his discovery of energy quanta."
- [1918 Nobel Prize in Physics] nobelprize.org

- ⚛ In 1905, Albert Einstein published a paper that advanced Planck's hypothesis, in which light energy is transported in 'quanta' to explain experimental data on the photoelectric effect. Einstein showed that light is a flow of photons.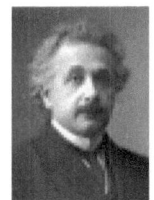
  - [albert einstein] [photoelectric effect] wikipedia

  - ⚛ *The 1921 Nobel Prize in Physics was awarded to Albert Einstein "for his services to Theoretical Physics, especially for his discovery of the law of the photoelectric effect".*
    - [1921 premio nobel de fisica] nobelprize.org

- ⚛ In 1910, Robert Millikan determined the magnitude of the electron's charge.
  - [robert millikan] [photoelectric effect] wikipedia

  - ⚛ *The 1923 Nobel Prize in Physics was awarded to Robert Andrews Millikan "for his work on the elementary charge of electricity and the photoelectric effect."*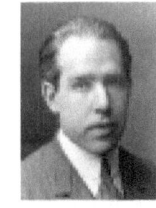
    - [1923 premio nobel de fisica] nobelprize.org

- ⚛ In 1913, Niels Bohr proposed in his model of the atom that electrons move around a nucleus, but only 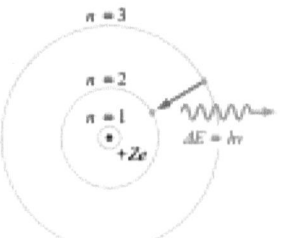 in prescribed orbits, and that if they jump to a lower energy orbit, they emit light of fixed wavelengths; this was incorporated into his theories about the 'quanta' of light.
  - [Niels Bohr] wikipedia

- *The 1922 Nobel Prize in Physics was awarded to Niels Henrik David Bohr "for his services in the investigation of the structure of atoms and the radiation emanating from them."*
    - [1922 Nobel Prize in Physics] nobelprize.org
- The photoelectric effect is the emission of electrons when electromagnetic radiation, such as light, strikes a material. The electrons emitted in this way are called photoelectrons.
    - [photoelectric effect] wikipedia

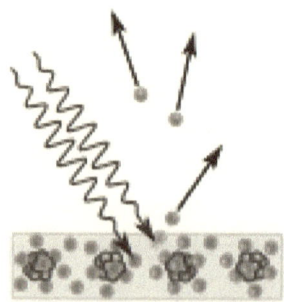

Fig. 20.1

- In the case of the eyes, when light hits the retina's photoreceptors, a flow of electrons is emitted, forming an electric current.

20.3 Visual center at the sensory level

- Visual phototransduction is the sensory transduction of the visual system, through which light is converted into electrical signals in the photoreceptor cells of the eye's retina.
    - [phototransduction] wikipedia

- ◆ *The 1967 Nobel Prize in Physiology or Medicine was awarded jointly to Ragnar Granit, Haldan Keffer Hartline, and George Wald "for their discoveries concerning the primary physiological and chemical visual processes of the eye."*
  - [1967 Nobel Prize in Physiology/Medicine] nobelprize.org
- ◆ The retina is the innermost, light-sensitive layer of tissue in the eye. The optics of the eye create a two-dimensional image of the visual world, focused on the retina, which translates it into nerve impulses to create visual perception in the brain. The retina serves a function analogous to that of film or the image sensor in a camera.
  - [retina] wikipedia

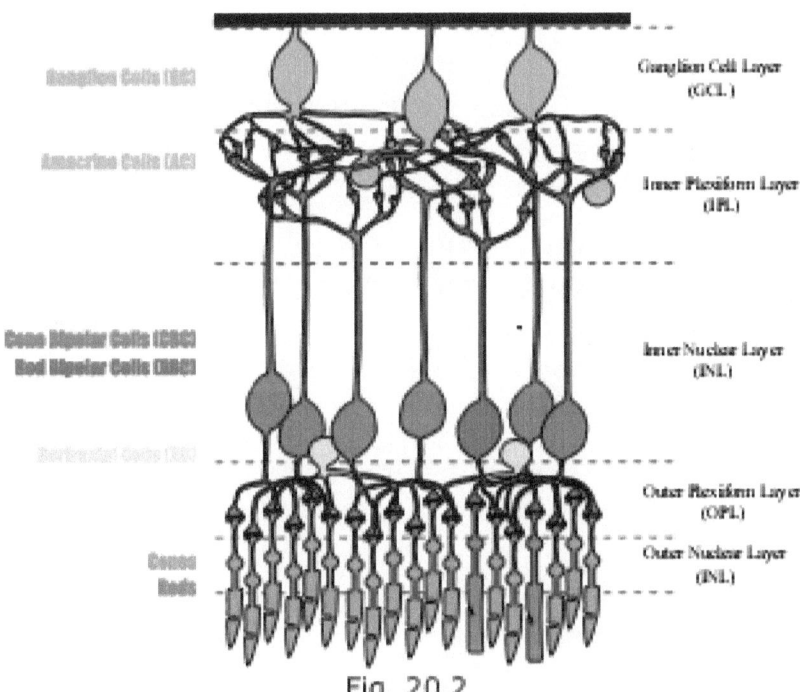

Fig. 20.2

- ◆ The figure shows in detail a cross-section of the different layers of neurons that make up the retina; networks of synapses interconnect the layers.
  - [cross section of the retina] wikipedia

- ⊕ At the neuronal level, the retina consists of the following layers of neurons: photoreceptors, horizontal, bipolar, amacrine, and ganglion:
  - [retina] wikipedia

1. ⊕ Photoreceptors: made up of rods, cones, and photosensitive ganglia.
   - [photoreceptors] wikipedia
     - ⊕ Rods: They detect peripheral visual information, are monochromatic (in the 498nm band), and function mainly in low light. There are about 96 million rods in each eye.
       - [rods] wikipedia
         - ⊕ Note: The speed of excitation response, between capture by the rods and detection in the visual center, is around 100 milliseconds, ten times slower than cones.
           - [rods vs cones] nature.com
     - ⊕ Cones: detect visual focus information in color and work in good lighting conditions. They are responsible for high-acuity vision, used in tasks such as reading. There are about 4.6 million cones in each eye.
       - [cones] wikipedia
         - ⊕ Note: The speed of excitation response, between capture by the cones and detection in the visual center, is around 10 milliseconds, ten times faster than rods.
           - [rods vs cones] nature.com
     - ⊕ Photosensitive ganglion cells: They detect information for the circadian rhythm, which determines the 24-hour cycle in the coordination of biological processes; they detect information for the pupillary reflex, which controls the opening of the iris;

And other things. In each eye, there are about 5,000 photosensitive ganglion cells.
- [photosensitive ganglion] [circadian rhythm] [pupillary reflex] wikipedia

- ◉ Note: Based on the above, we can establish that around 100 million photoreceptor cells capture visual information in each eye.
  - [cones] wikipedia

2. ◉ Horizontal: They integrate the information from several photoreceptors. Among their functions, they are believed to be responsible for increasing contrast and adapting to both bright and dim light conditions.
   - [horizontal] wikipedia

3. ◉ Bipolar: They act, directly or indirectly, to transmit signals from photoreceptors to ganglion cells.
   - [bipolar] wikipedia

4. ◉ Amacrines: detect direction and directional movement.
   - [amacrina] wikipedia

5. ◉ Ganglion: Their axons transmit all visual information to the center. Their axons form the optic nerve. Each eye has about a million ganglion cells; therefore, each optic nerve comprises a million axonal fibers.
   - [ganglionic] [optic nerve] wikipedia

   - ◉ Note: Given that, in each eye, there are about 100 million photoreceptor cells and that there are only one million ganglion cells to transmit visual information, then, on average, each ganglion cell converges the information of about 100 photoreceptors.

eduardo padilla-diaz

Thinking-1

◐ *"Initiation to its models. Interfacing the Visual and Motor Centers to a Thinker."*

21.1 Introduction

- ◈ Reflections on thinking (part 1):
- ◈ To understand thinking, we will present, in several parts, a series of models that incrementally cover it.
- ◐◈ Thinking is a set of mental processes controlled by the conscience, which determines what we will do in the immediate future after jointly analyzing the reality of the present, memories, future goals, and modulators such as emotions and affections. All of these concepts will be explained in greater detail later.
- ◐◈ To begin, we'll assume that Thinking works by executing a list of interrelated tasks, dedicating attention to each task for a very short time, and achieving apparent attention on all these tasks as if they were being attended to simultaneously.
- ◈ A straightforward proposal of how primitive thinking would operate is presented, opening the doors for us to begin to understand and comprehend how our thinking operates.

    1. ◈ Let us consider the example of a primitive thinking system (P-1), which uses a single processor to execute several tasks. It uses the visual information sensed by our eyes to see a white line (object of interest) painted in the middle of the road, which guides us to a

determined destination. P-1 will execute the following tasks cyclically: capture, analyze, and solve.

- ● Task 1 captures sensed visual information from our visual center to extract useful data, such as where we are about the white line.
- ● Task 2 analyzes the useful information extracted by Task 1 to achieve the following purpose: follow the white line painted on the road. If the white line appears in the center of the image, then we are on the correct course. If the white line appears to the left of the image, then the *thinker* has to correct the direction of our course to the right. If the white line appears to the right of the image, then the *thinker* must correct our course's direction to the left. If the line's color turns yellow, we must stop because we have reached the destination.
- ● Task 3 solve: According to the results of the analysis of Task 2, we must take a step forward in the given direction or stop if we have already reached the final destination.
- ● The following figure shows how the P-1 processor executes the three tasks sequentially and cyclically.

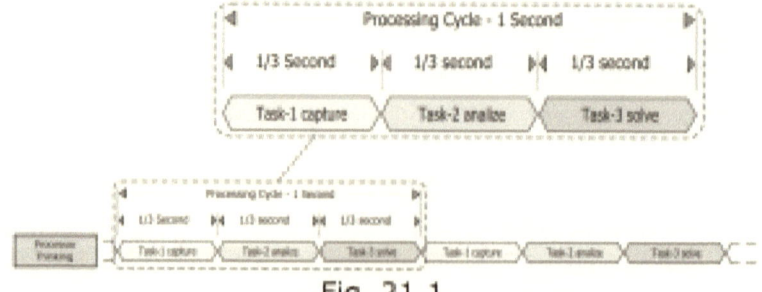

Fig. 21.1

If this P-1 devotes attention to each task for 1/3 of a second, then P-1 executes the three tasks sequentially and repeats them cyclically within each second.

- ⊕ The problem with this proposed P-1 processor is that it would be too limited to fulfill its function in terms of its processing capacity and the time it would have available to execute each task.

  - ⊕ Let's consider the case of Task 1, which is responsible for processing the visual context. To estimate the number of images/sec that Task 1 processes, we must consider that each eye simultaneously captures two concentric images: the ones under focus have 4.6 megapixels, captured at a 10ms rate, giving us 100 images/sec, while the ones surrounding those in focus have 92 megapixels captured at 100ms rate, giving us 10 images/sec. These gigantic megapixel figures show us that, to process video, a highly specialized processor must be dedicated to processing exclusively visual information to achieve this.

    - ⊕ A pixel is the smallest part of an image; it contains its color and intensity.

  - ⊕ Let us consider Task 2, which analyzes the useful information given by Task 1. This task's complexity depends on the complexity of the information it receives from Task 1 and the complexity of the information expected by Task 3. Task 2's complexity is thousands of times greater than that of Task 1.

  - ⊕ Let's consider the case of Task 3, which is in charge of moving the body step-by-step to follow the white line. The body's locomotor system comprises the skeleton, muscles, tendons, and other connective tissues. Our body has more than 650 skeletal muscles, each consisting of thousands of muscle fibers contracted by dozens of molecular robots of the myosin type. They contain spindle-type muscle sensors, which mainly detect changes in muscle length, and they have Golgi-type sensor tendons, which link the muscles to the bones and help control the maximum force each muscle can exert so that it does not break. Maintaining balance, or taking a step, requires hundreds of thousands of motor and monitoring microinstructions. Our mind is already equipped with innate locomotor knowledge that is responsible for relieving us of much of the complexity of the locomotor system. With all that, it takes us around six years to learn all the essential motor functions required to operate the body skillfully and safely in the environment. These complex functions show us that processing motor information, as such, requires a highly specialized processing system exclusively dedicated to processing the motor functions.

- [locomotor system] [myosin] [spindle] [golgi] wikipedia

2. Now, let's look at a second model of P-1, which is much more efficient than the previous one since it uses three processors that operate in parallel.

   a. Processor #1: We will call this processor the thinker, which will be dedicated to processing only what is related to thinking.

   b. Processor #2: We will add a processor exclusively dedicated to processing the sensations produced by the different light sources present in the visual field. Let's call this processor the Visual Center.

      - The Visual Center will perform several functions on various information channels, but we will only use the Reality and MP channels for now.

- ⊕ The Reality channel receives the visual field we capture with our eyes. It projects it internally in a mental image that allows us to feel it continuously with excellent resolution.
- ⊕ The MP channel (thinking messages) looks for the new image's white line (object of interest). It extracts its position and other attributes, and if there are changes, it packs them into a photogram that is sent to the thinking center for processing.
  - ⊕ Photograms contain useful visual information. The next book in this series, titled: 'The Width of the Present,' includes the chapter Thinking Messages, where the photograms are described in more detail.

c. ⊕ Processor #3: We will also add another processor dedicated exclusively to processing the motor context. We are going to call this processor the Motor Center. This processor will perform two very important functions:

- ⊕ Move our body with very high skill. The Motor Center receives internal orders that determine which foot is anchored, which foot takes the step, maintains the balance of the body, and a countless number of motor functions that are carried out automatically so that it moves harmoniously regardless of what we are thinking.
  - ⊕ Later, we will see that if something unexpected happens while we move, such as tripping, our Motor Center resorts to reflexes to resolve these cases immediately and automatically and then informs our conscience of what happened.

- ◆ When the *thinker* tells the Motor Center to take a step, it only has to issue a high-level command, which we will call a motogram, that indicates the direction and distance of the step. The Motor Center takes the command, issues hundreds of thousands of motor microinstructions, and reads hundreds of thousands of monitoring signals to carry out what is ordered gracefully and without losing balance. In the example, the thinker can also give the Motor Center commands to decrease or increase the step's speed or stop walking.

d. ◆ With the addition of the two processors to the second model, the *thinker* will have more time to process what we think. So, we will have to make a time adjustment in the previous model of P-1.

- ◆ The following figure shows a timing diagram of the three processors and the times of the thinker's tasks. As can be seen, the thinker's active time was considerably reduced.

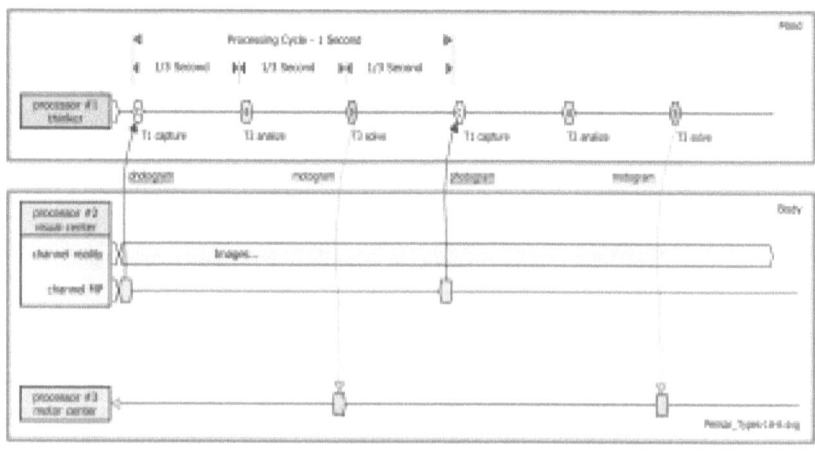

Fig. 21.2

- ◆ Let's see how the times spent on the thinker's tasks were reduced with the addition of the Visual Center and Motor Center processors:

- ◈ Task 1: The thinker receives a much more compact and efficient photogram from the Visual Center. The photogram starts this task. The time this task spends fulfilling its function is reduced from 333ms to less than 10ms.
- ◈ Task 2: no longer has to analyze the perceived visual information in its native form, which is very complex and extensive. Task 2 analyzes the content of the photogram, which is simple and compact and contains information about the object of interest in the image. The photogram simplifies tracking the white line painted on the road until reaching the destination. The time spent by Task 2 to fulfill its function is reduced from 333ms to less than 10ms.
- ◈ Task 3 no longer has to spend time issuing hundreds of thousands of motor microinstructions and reading hundreds of thousands of monitoring signals to move the body - step-by-step - in a graceful way without losing balance. Task 3 only sends the motor center a motogram containing a high-level command indicating the direction and distance of the step. The motogram is compact and efficient, so the motor center is autonomously responsible for taking the step. The time spent by Task 3 commanding the motor center is reduced from 333ms to less than 10ms.
- ◈ Note: In humans, it has been found experimentally that an auditory signal can reach the central processing mechanisms in 8 to 10 ms. In comparison, the visual stimulus takes around 20 to 40 ms.
  - [mental chronometry] wikipedia
- ◈ Since the total time P-1 now spends executing its tasks has been reduced from 1 second to about 30 ms, P-1 could reduce the time it spends on each cycle from 1 second to 30 ms to execute about 30 cycles per second,

instead of one cycle per second. But this cannot be done yet, as long as we do not change how to handle the motor commands that take many times longer to execute than the thinking cycle lasts.

- ● This second model is better than the first. However, it still needs to be feasible since the execution of the motor commands is variable in duration, typically taking around 500 to 1500 ms when we take a step.

- ● Now, let's look at a third P-1 model that is more feasible since it can process motor commands that allow us to take steps of variable duration, typically from 500 to 1500 ms. The following figure shows the timing diagram of this new model. The changes are explained below:

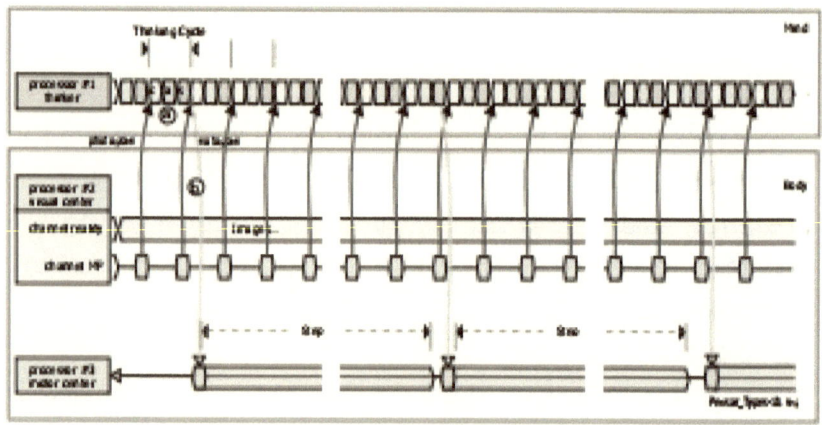

Fig. 21.3

a. ● The *thinker* executes his three tasks of capturing, analyzing, and solving, one after the other, all with the help of the conscience.

b. ● In this model of the thinker, the solving task only sends motor commands when the Motor Center is not busy.

c. ● As a new image arrives, the Visual Center projects it into the Reality channel. It draws the thinker's attention by sending a photogram, which forces the execution of a new thinking cycle.

d. ⊕ The thinking cycle allows the thinker to understand the previously projected image.

- ⊕ The next book, The Width of the Present, presents a more advanced thinking model that can process several thoughts, handle multiple sources of visual attention, anticipate the immediate future, and much more.

Epilog 1

- *Thematics of the next book in the series: The Width of the Present.*

0. [Cover-2] *The Width of the Present - Book 2 of the series: Modeling the Body-Mind.*
1. [TOC] *Thematics and Exploration Plan.*
2. [Conventions] *Considerations about revisions, references, TOCs, and Epilogs.*
3. [Abstract 2] *Quantum Thinking Physics is the discrete information framework consciousness uses.*
4. [Serialization] *The most crucial transformer in understanding and exchanging our thoughts.*
5. [Data Structures] *Matter dwells in an undetermined probability state without structuring.*
6. [Width of the Present] *Paradox used by the conscience to insert itself in the domain of time.*
7. [Time Segments] *They only exist in the mind to give us access to the present, past, and future.*
8. [BioBots] *These wonderful beings inhabit our body from the molecular to the multi-organic rings.*
9. [Molecular Nets] *The intracellular networks where molecular robots operate.*
10. [Neural Nets] *Neurons connect reality, virtuality, and modulators with body and mind so we can be.*
11. [Bot Nets] *Networks where cellular robots circulate to transport supplies, repair, and protect.*
12. [Signaling] *Signals used in the neural and cellular networks to exert actions in cells.*
13. [Memories-2] *These operational memories store the innate, immediate, and acquired knowledge.*
14. [Knowledge] *It is where we store what we know to help us decide what to do next.*
15. [Issues] *Gradual conscient activities processed by thinkers at the thinking center.*
16. [Channels] *Stream useful information from sensory centers to thinkers and motor centers.*

17. [Entanglement] *How the object of interest under focus entangles with thinking and consciousness.*
18. [Quantumness] *The fabric of quantum thinking physics: a paradigm for modeling consciousness.*
19. [VC-2] *Visual Center 2: Automatic detection of object attributes, reflexes handling, and more.*
20. [MC-2] *Motor Center 2: Locomotion, balance, movement fuidity, precision, reflexes, command interface.*
21. [Thinking Messages] *Sensory informatics paradigm bridges changes and states to the thinking system.*
22. [Thinking-2] *Quantum thinking in all thinkers, attention arbitration, anticipacion, and more.*
23. [Awareness] *Is the state of conscious comprehension of all thinking and feeling of all sensations.*
24. [Epilog-2] *Thematics of the next book in the series: Tokens and Words.*
25. [Copyrights] *List of copyright certificates that protect these works.*
26. [Dedication] *To my children: Mariana, Andres, and Camilo.*
27. [Back-cover-2] *Brief about the author Eduardo Padilla-Diaz and his works.*

eduardo padilla-diaz

Copyrights

List of copyright certificates that protect these works:

Entity	Title	Copyright Certificate	Date
Colombian Ministry of Interior	Ancho del Presente	10-1142-210	Jul 1, 2023
Colombian Ministry of Interior	Anillos de la Mente	10-1152-391	Aug 10, 2023
Colombian Ministry of Interior	Ancho del Presente	10-1170-247	Oct 24, 2023
Colombian Ministry of Interior	Rings of the Mind	10-1178-253	Nov 30, 2023
Colombian Ministry of Interior	Awareness	10-1204-369	Apr 10, 2024
Colombian Ministry of Interior	Quantumness	10-1204-416	Apr 10, 2024
Colombian Ministry of Interior	Entanglement	10-1205-1	Apr 10, 2024
Colombian Ministry of Interior	Time Segments	10-1205-2	Apr 10, 2024

eduardo padilla-diaz

Dedication

To my children: Mariana, Andres, and Camilo.

eduardo padilla-diaz

Rings of the Mind

eduardo padilla-diaz

Rings of the Mind

www.ingramcontent.com/pod-product-compliance
Lightning Source LLC
Chambersburg PA
CBHW031920240526
45464CB00021B/611